D0441584

NORTHERN NEW MEXICO
NORTH CENTRAL CAMPGROUNDS:
CARSON NATIONAL FOREST
1. CANJILON LAKES CAMPGROUND
2. CHACO CANYON CAMPGROUND
3. JICARILLA APACHE LAKE CAMPGROUND
4. HOPEWELL LAKE CAMPGROUND

NORTHEAST CAMPGROUNDS:
CARSON NATIONAL FOREST
5. COLUMBINE CAMPGROUND
6. ELEPHANT ROCK CAMPGROUND
7. FAWN LAKES CAMPGROUND
8. JUNE BUG CAMPGROUND
9. COYOTE CREEK STATE PARK CAMPGROUND
10. MORPHY LAKE STATE PARK CAMPGROUND
11. SUGARITE CANYON STATE PARK CAMPGROUND
12. VALLE VIDAL CAMPGROUNDS

NORTH CENTRAL CAMPGROUNDS: SANTA FE NATIONAL FOREST (JEMEZ AND CUBA AREA)
13. SAN ANTONIO CAMPGROUND
14. REDONDO CAMPGROUND
15. JEMEZ FALLS CAMPGROUND
16. BANDELIER NATIONAL MONUMENT CAMPGROUND
17. FENTON LAKE STATE PARK CAMPGROUND
18. CLEAR CREEK CAMPGROUND
19. RIO DE LAS VACAS CAMPGROUND

NORTH CENTRAL CAMPGROUNDS: SANTA FE NATIONAL FOREST (SANTA FE, PECOS, LAS VEGAS AREA)
20. BLACK CANYON CAMPGROUND
21. FIELD TRACT CAMPGROUND
22. HOLY GHOST CAMPGROUND
23. IRON GATE CAMPGROUND
24. JACKS CREEK CAMPGROUND
25. VILLANUEVA STATE PARK CAMPGROUND
26. COCHITI LAKE CAMPGROUND

CENTRAL NEW MEXICO
MANZANO AREA
27. CAPILLA PEAK CAMPGROUND
28. NEW CANYON CAMPGROUND
29. MANZANO MOUNTAINS STATE PARK CAMPGROUND
30. RED CANYON CAMPGROUND

TAJIQUE AREA
31. FOURTH OF JULY CAMPGROUND
32. TAJIQUE CAMPGROUND

SOUTHERN NEW MEXICO
SOUTH CENTRAL STATE PARKS
33. CABALLO LAKE STATE PARK CAMPGROUND
34. PERCHA DAM STATE PARK CAMPGROUND
35. AGUIRRE SPRING CAMPGROUND
36. PANCHO VILLA STATE PARK CAMPGROUND

NORTHERN GILA
37. WATER CANYON CAMPGROUND
38. DATIL WELL CAMPGROUND
39. PINON CAMPGROUND
40. JUNIPER CAMPGROUND
41. DIPPING VAT AT SNOW LAKE CAMPGROUND

SOUTHERN GILA
42. IRON CREEK CAMPGROUND
43. CITY OF ROCKS STATE PARK CAMPGROUND
44. GILA CLIFF DWELLINGS NATIONAL MONUMENT CAMPGROUND
45. LAKE ROBERTS CAMPGROUND

LINCOLN
46. VALLEY OF FIRES CAMPGROUND
47. OAKGROVE CAMPGROUND
48. SOUTHFORK CAMPGROUND
49. SILVER LAKE CAMPGROUND
50. PINES CAMPGROUND

Other titles in this series

The Best in Tent Camping: The Carolinas
The Best in Tent Camping: Colorado
The Best in Tent Camping: Florida
The Best in Tent Camping: Georgia
The Best in Tent Camping: Maryland
The Best in Tent Camping: Minnesota
The Best in Tent Camping: Missouri and the Ozarks
The Best in Tent Camping: Montana
The Best in Tent Camping: New England
The Best in Tent Camping: New Jersey
The Best in Tent Camping: New Mexico
The Best in Tent Camping: New York State
The Best in Tent Camping: Northern California
The Best in Tent Camping: Oregon
The Best in Tent Camping: Pennsylvania
The Best in Tent Camping: The Southern Appalachian and Smoky Mountains
The Best in Tent Camping: Southern California
The Best in Tent Camping: Tennessee and Kentucky
The Best in Tent Camping: Virginia
The Best in Tent Camping: Washington
The Best in Tent Camping: West Virginia
The Best in Tent Camping: Wisconsin

THE BEST IN TENT CAMPING

A GUIDE FOR CAR CAMPERS WHO HATE RVs,
CONCRETE SLABS, AND LOUD PORTABLE STEREOS

NEW MEXICO

MONTE R. PARR

MENASHA RIDGE PRESS
BIRMINGHAM, ALABAMA

*This book is lovingly dedicated to my lovely wife, Susan Sherwood Parr.
Thank you for all the encouragement and support,
and especially our adventures in the wilderness together.*

Copyright © 2008 by Monte R. Parr
All rights reserved
Printed in the United States of America
Published by Menasha Ridge Press
Distributed by Publishers Group West
First edition, first printing

   Printed on recycled paper

Library of Congress Cataloging-in-Publication Data

Parr, Monte R.
    Best in tent camping, New Mexico : a guide for campers who hate RVs,
    concrete slabs, and loud portable stereos / by Monte R. Parr.
        p. cm.
    Includes bibliographical references and index.
    ISBN-13: 978-0-89732-602-5 (alk. paper)
    ISBN-10: 0-89732-602-4 (alk. paper)
        1. Camp sites, facilities, etc.—New Mexico—Directories. 2. Camping—New
    Mexico—Guidebooks. 3. New Mexico—Guidebooks. I. Title.
    GV191.42.N6P37 2008
    917.8906'854—dc22

                              2007049419

Cover and text design by Ian Szymkowiak, Palace Press International, Inc.
Cover photo by David L. Moore / Alamy
Cartography by Steve Jones, Jennie Zehmer and Monte R. Parr

Menasha Ridge Press
P.O. Box 43673
Birmingham, Alabama 35243
www.menasharidge.com

TABLE OF CONTENTS

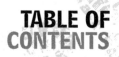

NORTHERN NEW MEXICO 19

NORTH CENTRAL CAMPGROUNDS: CARSON NATIONAL FOREST

NORTHEAST CAMPGROUNDS: CARSON NATIONAL FOREST

NORTH CENTRAL CAMPGROUNDS: SANTA FE NATIONAL FOREST
JEMEZ AND CUBA AREA

NORTH CENTRAL CAMPGROUNDS: SANTA FE NATIONAL FOREST
SANTA FE, PECOS, LAS VEGAS AREA

ACKNOWLEDGMENTS

I WISH TO EXPRESS the deepest heartfelt gratitude to the following people for their love, kindness, support, encouragement, and friendships: my wife Susan Sherwood Parr; dear stepson Chris Livingston; brother Robert and Debra Parr; daughter Kimmie Parr; grandchildren Paige and Austin; my dear mom-in-law, Neriede Sherwood, and the entire Sherwood family. Special thanks to my dear friend R. D. "Don" Eiler, host at Jemez Falls Campground. Don has been a godsend with his vast knowledge of New Mexico's wildlands.

My dear friends and spiritual mentors, Pastor Skip and Lenya Heitzig, and Pastor Eric and Debbie Larson. Thanks to Chip Lusko, Peter Benson, and Steve Reimann at KNKT 707.1 Connection Radio for their interest in my projects and for airtime. Special thanks to Jicarilla Apache Chief Reynard Faber for his warmth and long-time friendship.

I sincerely wish to thank Russell Helms, Molly Merkle, and all the kind folks at Menasha Ridge Press for their input, professional skills, and encouragement. They have no idea what an adventure they have given me. I am grateful and humbled to be chosen as the author for this book.

I would like to express my gratitude to the members of the following government agencies. These folks were friendly, helpful, and informative. Without their assistance, this project could not have been completed:

**Jicarilla Apache Nation • Mescalero Apache Nation • National Park Service
New Mexico County Sheriff's Departments • New Mexico Fish and Wildlife
New Mexico State Parks • New Mexico State Police
United States Army Corps of Engineers • United States Bureau of Land Management
United States Fish And Wildlife Service • United States Forest Service**

I would like to thank the following businesses for their help and inspiration with this project:

**Amanda's General Store • Der Markt Grocery • Manzano Tiendita • Ray's General Store
Sportsmen's Warehouse • The Sherwood Company • Word Productions**

I would like to thank the following manufacturers for their excellent quality products used while researching this project:

**Apple Computers • Bushnell Optics • Coleman tents, coolers, lanterns, stoves, and sleeping bags • Dell Computers • Delorme Topographic Maps • Eureka Tents • Ford Motor Company
Garmin GPS Systems • Kelty Sleeping Bags • Meade Optics
National Geographic Topographic Maps • Nikon Cameras • Sony Cameras • Olympus Optics
Winchester Knives • Yamaha Motorcycle**

PREFACE

I HAVE LOVED THE OUTDOORS since I was knee high to a short toad. I was raised by my grandparents, who taught me to slow down, be observant, and appreciate the gifts Mother Nature has generously given all of us. I was like most kids; I started camping in the backyard, with a sheet draped over the clothesline, sleeping on an old army cot and sleeping bag. In high school, I spent many hours hiking the hundreds of acres of hardwood forests behind our home with a knapsack, sleeping bag, and an old Army pup tent.

My early adult life was spent backpacking and car camping the wonderful state parks throughout Nebraska. I moved to Colorado for two years and continued backpacking and car camping the high country. I moved to New Mexico in August of 1988, and the next weekend I launched my first trip into the Jemez wilderness. It was there that I discovered the "Land of Enchantment" was where I was destined to be.

I am convinced that tent camping is the purest and most rewarding method of experiencing nature. During high winds, drenching downpours, and lightning storms, tent camping is a challenge; but I prefer a tent any day to sleeping in a metal box. On a brightly moonlit night, I love the shadows of the tree branches dancing on the roof of the tent. I love to watch the campfire flames and glowing embers. I love going to sleep with the sounds of a night bird calling, the hooting of an owl from deep in the forest, and the distant howl of the coyote.

I love the sounds of the mountain breeze as it catches the upper branches of a giant ponderosa—wind gusting through ponderosa pine trees, sounds like the ocean surf rushing to the shore, rising then cascading, and then rising again. You can hear the creaking of the branches. You watch the camber of the tree as it bends in the wind.

It is a healthy choice to escape the electronic paraphernalia that inundates our society and all the stresses that come with technology. I leave the gadgets at home. It seems the simpler you camp, the more you enjoy the experience. When I started camping, I used an old saucepan and a roll of foil and cooked like a cowboy. When I bought a cookstove and lantern, I thought I was in hog heaven!

When I began this project, I had absolutely no clue what a delightful undertaking it would be. This opportunity has allowed me to visit every county in New Mexico, every national forest, and all of the major historical areas the 47th state offers. I traveled in excess of 9,000 miles, and the traveling allowed me to camp more than 30 weekends in 2007, which in and of itself was an absolute blast. I visited more than 160 campgrounds. The majority of them deserve a profile in this book; eliminating many deserving campgrounds was difficult, but inevitable.

It is my sincere wish that this book will enhance your camping experiences in New Mexico, and that you experience all the joys and blessings in your travels that I have had.

Respectfully,
Monte R. Parr

ABOUT THE AUTHOR

MONTE **R. PARR'S OUTDOOR INTERESTS** were inspired as a child by his grand-parents and treks into the San Bernardino Mountains of Southern California. His high school years were spent hiking and camping the hardwood forests behind his family home in Iowa. Monte has lived in California, Iowa, Nebraska, Mississippi, Colorado, and New Mexico.

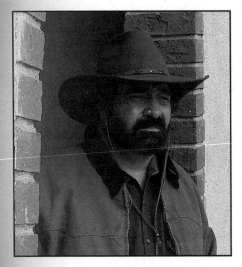

Monte is experienced in backpacking, back-country motorcycle camping, and cross-country ski and snowshoe camping. He has camped extensively throughout Iowa, Nebraska, Colorado, Wyoming, and New Mexico.

Monte is an accomplished photographer with interests including astronomy, hiking, mountain biking, and fishing. Monte's fascination with Old West history has taken him to dozens of ghost towns, old military outposts, and many ancient Native American cliff dwellings and ruins throughout New Mexico and Arizona. Monte is a U.S. Air Force veteran; he worked as a ground crew member on C-130 Air-craft and is an avid military aircraft historian.

Monte's writing projects include his first book, *Adventures in Camping,* published by Word Productions, Inc. He is also a lyricist and poet, publishing his works on a Web site still under development, **montesoldwest.com.** He has recently created "Monte's Old West Chuckwagon Spice," a tantalizing barbecue spice, and is currently working on many recipes for camping.

Since moving to New Mexico in 1988, Monte has logged more than 800 nights under the stars, experiencing mountain, desert, and canyon camping, in every county in New Mexico. He has been a regular guest on the radio program ABQ-Connect for the past three years.

Monte is an accounts consultant for a major communications company in Albu-querque, New Mexico. His wife, Susan Parr, an accomplished author, and dogs Sheppie, Steffie, and Rascal join him frequently on his journeys.

INTRODUCTION

WELCOME TO NEW MEXICO, THE LAND OF ENCHANTMENT! Our beloved state is a diverse land of contrasts—of canyons, deserts, mesas, high mountains, rivers, lakes, and glorious sunsets. This is a magnificent state in which to experience the best in tent camping.

New Mexico is the fifth largest state in the nation, with 121,655 square miles of land mass. Our population ranks 36th in the nation, with under 2 million people. The population density is slightly less than 15 people per square mile, in which it ranks 45th.

The mountains of New Mexico aren't as high as neighboring Colorado's peaks, but our mountains are as breathtaking as any on the planet. Wheeler Peak, at 13,161 feet, is the highest of six summits above 13,000 feet. There are 32 peaks over 12,000 feet, and 37 mountains tower over 11,000 feet.

New Mexico has five managed national forests: Carson, Santa Fe, Cibola, Gila, and Lincoln. The Bureau of Land Management has divided New Mexico into seven field offices to manage public lands: Farmington, Rio Puerco, Socorro, Las Cruces, Taos, Roswell, and Carlsbad. New Mexico features 34 state parks with a diverse landscape of lakes, mountains, canyons, forests, deserts, and historical sites. More than 30 hot springs scattered throughout the state attract many naturalists (with and without bathing attire), and many of these hot springs are located near campgrounds. Without question, you will find dozens of campgrounds you will wish to revisit.

Often you will spot elk herds numbering in the hundreds grazing in high-country grasslands. Also look for mountain lions, bobcats, black bears, mule deer, buffalo, pronghorn antelope, coyotes, Mexican gray wolves, javelinas, and ringtail cats—just a few species of wildlife native to our state.

The bird population in New Mexico is enormous, with more species than most birdwatchers can identify. The Rio Grande River Valley south of Socorro, New Mexico, is on the migratory flyway, and several protected waterfowl habitats are nearby. We are blessed with a large population of hummingbirds, so you might want to bring a feeder; they are delightful little visitors to your camp and easy to photograph.

Canyon walls rise dramatically from valley floors, providing breeding habitat for bald and golden eagles, various species of hawks, and the endangered peregrine falcon. Mesa walls tell the geologic history of this state with exposed stratum of rock, lava, clay, and sandstone in colorful contrasts that cannot be described in words. Some mesa walls are painted green, with pinon, juniper, and cedar trees clinging to their steep sides.

Every spring the cacti bloom in vibrant colors under the bright Chihuahuan desert sun. Knee-high silver sage paints the desert floor with a silvery green landscape. Beautiful yucca plant stalks bloom with shoots filled with white flowers. Greasewood, creosote, and mesquite trees are common throughout the desert. In the mountains, wildflowers of every color explode in springtime and stay until frost appears in the fall.

Arroyos fill with rainwater and pour over the parched land as the monsoon season arrives in July. The thirsty deserts and Sangre De Cristo Mountains drink in the moisture and become lush and green. The increase in precipitation over the past two years has made New Mexico greener than native residents have seen in their lifetime.

In autumn, aspen, oak, cottonwood, and willow trees explode in bright oranges, yellows, and reds, painting the mountains, valleys, and river basins.

Winter snows begin in November. Skiers arrive at the slopes and resorts dotting the state. Snowbirds escaping the harsh winters of the northern states also arrive in November across the southern half of New Mexico. They feed the economies of dozens of towns through the month of April.

South of Truth or Consequences, New Mexico, the Mesilla (pronounced Meh–SEE–yuh) Valley is a glorious contrast of green adjacent to the brown Turtle and Caballo mountains to the east and brown desert to the west. The Mesilla Valley follows the Rio Grand River from north of Hatch, New Mexico, all the way south to El Paso, Texas. Since the valley is quite fertile, agriculture is the primary activity in this area. Just about every vegetable you can imagine is grown here, notably the Vidalia and Mayan sweet onions. The world's largest pecan orchard is located in the valley, and the area is famous for its pistachio nuts. Fruit orchards produce apples, peaches, plums, and other fruit. And the world-famous New Mexico green and red chiles are grown here and shipped worldwide.

Many geologic wonders abound in New Mexico: Tent Rocks, La Ventana Arch, Echo Amphitheatre, Valley of Fires, Chimney Rock, Carlsbad Caverns, and the Taos Gorge are just a few. Six state and 13 national monuments provide diverse educational, historical, and cultural experiences. Bandalier National Monument, Jemez State Monument, Chaco Canyon, and Gila Cliff Dwellings National Monument are just a few of the historic sites New Mexico offers. Due to constant attacks by nomadic bands of Apache, New Mexico was protected by 18 permanent forts and many more temporary cavalry camps. Six of the cavalry posts were home to Buffalo Soldiers.

Rock hounds keep busy in New Mexico year-round, attracted by quartz, turquoise, and dozens of other minerals. Many old mines dot the state and provide fascinating tales of wild and rowdy boomtowns that quickly became ghost towns as the gold and silver strikes played out. New Mexico is rich in history. If you love the Old West, we have a wild and wooly experience waiting for you. Dozens of crumbling ghost towns await your discovery.

Fort Sumner is the final resting place of Billy the Kid. West of Ruidoso, New Mexico, you'll find the sight of the Lincoln County Wars and the home and grave of Smokey the Bear. New Mexico has two Civil War battlefields: Glorieta Pass and Valverde. Visit the historic border town of Columbus and retrace the steps of Pancho Villa's army as they perpetrated the famous raid in 1916.

New Mexico has the largest Native American population in the nation, with more than 134,000 people. Twenty-two different tribal lands provide many diverse camping, hunting, fishing, hiking, and other recreational opportunities.

New Mexico is also the land of Spanish conquistadors. You can walk the same paths as Coronado, Sanchez, Chamuscado, Rodriguez, Gallegos, Espejo, Sosa, and De Onate as they went searching for the treasures of the seven cities of Cibola.

Numerous cattle trails await your exploration. If you're a railroad buff, the rich history of the Atchison, Topeka, and Santa Fe Railroad expansion of the 1800s might interest you. You can camp near the birthplace of the great Apache warrior Geronimo in the Gila River Valley and explore the same trails and hideouts used by Geronimo, Cochise, Mangas Coloradas, and Victorio, who evaded capture for 25 years.

Hundreds of miles of equestrian trails offer the delight of a trail ride or camping on horseback. If you enjoy backcountry camping, check out the endless opportunities available to backpackers. Off-road motorcycle and all-terrain-vehicle trails lead to remote wild country where few venture. Check for laws regarding off-road vehicle use—new laws were enacted in 2006.

New Mexico is a land of deep forests, every bit as lovely as the other Rocky Mountain states. Because the Southern Rockies are generally more arid than the mountain states to the north, New Mexico is susceptible to extreme fire danger. Over the past few years, the state has been blessed with wonderful amounts of rainfall, but during dry periods, the forests can become a lethal tinderbox in a short period of time. In the 1980s through the early 2000s, we experienced severe drought resulting in forest closures. When we experience a dry spell, be prepared to camp without a campfire. Stage II restrictions (no campfires) may go into effect with little warning, but camp stoves are still allowed. Camping during Stage II fire restrictions is a delightful experience because the campgrounds are less crowded and the fragrances of the forests are indescribable.

So, bienvenidos! Welcome to our state!

THE OVERVIEW MAP AND OVERVIEW-MAP KEY

Use the overview map on the inside front cover to assess the exact location of each campground. The campground's number appears not only on the overview map but also on the map key facing the overview map, in the table of contents, and on the profile's first page.

The book is organized by region, as indicated in the table of contents. A map legend that details the symbols found on the campground layout maps appears on the inside back cover.

CAMPGROUND-LAYOUT MAPS

Each profile contains a detailed campground-layout map that provides an overhead look at campground sites, internal roads, facilities, and other key items. Each campground entrance's GPS coordinates are included with each profile.

GPS COORDINATES

This book also includes GPS coordinates for each campground profile in two formats: Universal Transverse Mercator (UTM) and latitude–longitude. Latitude–longitude coordinates tell you where you are by locating a point west (latitude) of the 0° meridian line that passes through Greenwich, England, and north or south of the 0° (longitude) line that belts the Earth, aka the equator.

Topographic maps show latitude and longitude as well as UTM grid lines. Known as UTM coordinates, the numbers index a specific point using a grid method. The survey datum used to arrive at the coordinates in this book is WGS84 (versus NAD27 or WGS83). For readers who own a GPS unit, whether handheld or onboard a vehicle, the latitude–longitude or UTM coordinates may be entered into the GPS unit (just make sure your unit is set to navigate using WGS84 datum). Now you can navigate directly to the campground. (Coordinates that do not lead directly to a campground entrance, such as those for a general state-park entrance or a boat landing, have been noted as such.)

That said, however, readers can easily find all campgrounds in this book by using the directions given and the campground layout map, which shows at least one major road leading into the area. But for those who enjoy using the latest GPS technology to navigate, the necessary data have been provided. A brief explanation of the UTM coordinates for Chaco Canyon Campground (page 23), follows:

UTM Zone (WGS84) 13S
Easting 0239140
Northing 3991414
Latitude N 36 01'56.4"
Longitude W 107 53' 42.5"

The UTM zone number 13 refers to one of the 60 vertical zones of the Universal Transverse Mercator (UTM) projection. Each zone is 6 degrees wide. The UTM zone letter *S* refers to one of the 20 horizontal zones that span from 80 degrees South to 84 degrees North. The easting number 0239140 indicates in meters how far east or west a point is from the central meridian of the zone. Increasing easting coordinates on a topographic map or on your GPS screen indicate that you are moving east; decreasing easting coordinates indicate you are moving west. The northing number 3991414 references in meters how far you are from the equator. Above and below the equator, increasing northing coordinates indicate you are traveling north; decreasing northing coordinates indicate you are traveling south.

To learn more about how to enhance your outdoor experiences with GPS technology, refer to *GPS Outdoors: A Practical Guide for Outdoor Enthusiasts* (Menasha Ridge Press).

THE CAMPGROUND PROFILE

In addition to maps, each profile contains a concise but informative narrative of the campground, as well as individual sites. This descriptive text is enhanced with four helpful sidebars: Ratings, Key Information, Getting There (accurate driving directions that lead you to the campground from the nearest major roadway), and GPS Coordinates. On the first page of each profile is a Ratings box.

RATING SYSTEM

Each campground is rated from one to five stars. It was genuinely difficult to choose certain campgrounds and exclude others; I made my choices objectively so as to select the camps that best serve tent campers.

BEAUTY I love high-country camping, but wide-open desert camping has a beauty that everyone should experience. One case in point was a camping trip to Caballo Lake State Park, a desert lake. It was a warm summer evening, and the clouds on the western horizon painted the skyline with phenomenal pinks, reds, and oranges. The Caballo Mountains to my east, across the Rio Grande River, turned a blazing fiery red. Later that night, the wide-open sky was a myriad of the brightest stars.

The sunsets New Mexico is famous for aren't always as visible in the mountains, and because of the forest canopy, stargazing is limited. Depending on the exact location, forest campgrounds may provide or obscure incredible views. New Mexico lakes are awesome at sunset. On a windless night, the moon and stars reflect off the water and create a joyful experience.

PRIVACY Some campgrounds are just poorly designed. I'll tell you if campsites are spaced too closely for reasonable comfort. When camping beside a river, expect some inevitable intrusion by anglers.

SPACIOUSNESS Space is an important commodity for the tent camper. Newer campgrounds tend to compact sites, while older established campgrounds provide more leg room. I did not mention the most spacious campsite numbers. Almost all campgrounds profiled in this book are on a first-come, first-serve basis, and the best sites may be occupied already. I did mention sites that could be considered honeymoon suites.

QUIET Nothing is more lovely than the sound of the night wind in the pines, the creaking of a 100-foot-tall ponderosa, or a rushing mountain stream. And nothing is more obnoxious than radios, barking dogs, and generators running full bore all day long. Noise management is the responsibility of every camper. Most campground hosts are either unwilling or unable to enforce the serenity of a campground; and law enforcement officers often have bigger fish to fry than loud radios.

RVs will be at some of the campgrounds I have profiled; they have been a part of the wilderness equation since they were invented. However, it seems many former RV owners are rediscovering tent camping. When camping near RVs, set your tent back away from the busy areas of the camp for increased privacy.

SECURITY Every camper deserves a safe environment. I have never experienced pilferage from my campsite, but I take precautions, and I make some recommendations concerning security throughout this book. I will note if a campground host is on-site and comment on law-enforcement patrols. Most campgrounds I profile will have excellent security, but some have little to none. If the campground is isolated, there are fewer visitors. I rarely have to carry a weapon, but I do in isolated areas.

Wild parties have become rare at established campgrounds. The U.S. Forest Service has become intolerant of revelries, and New Mexico State Parks have nearly eliminated the problem. I applaud the zero-tolerance policy.

CLEANLINESS Cleanliness is a priority for all campers. Keeping the camp clean for others is a responsibility we should all take seriously. The forest service and campground hosts need our help in maintaining pristine camps.

I will comment on building conditions and facility provisions such as restrooms, water quality, fireplace and picnic tables, parking, road conditions, and dense vegetation overgrowth and weed management. If a campground falls below reasonable sanitary expectations, I will tell you why I rated it the way I did.

LIFE ZONES OF NEW MEXICO

LOWER SONORAN

To 4,500 feet

Temperature and evaporation high, precipitation low.

CHARACTERISTIC PLANTS:

Mesquite, creosote, greasewood, yucca, agave, four wing saltbrush, native grasses.

CHARACTERISTIC ANIMALS:

Coatamundi, javelina, ringtail cat, desert bighorn sheep, coyote, mountain lion, rattlesnake, lizards, box turtle.

UPPER SONORAN

4,500 feet to 7,500 feet

Temperature modest to high, evaporation high, precipitation modest.

CHARACTERISTIC PLANTS:

Alligator juniper, chihuahua pine, chamisa, cholla, apache plume, gambel oak, box elder, salt cedar, cottonwood, pinon, juniper, red cedar.

CHARACTERISTIC ANIMALS:

White-tailed deer, mule deer, pronghorn antelope, black bear, prairie dog, rabbit.

TRANSITION

7,500 feet to 8,200 feet

Milder summer, cold winter, substantial rain and snow, evaporation modest.

CHARACTERISTIC PLANTS:

Ponderosa, limber, and apache pine, mountain maple, New Mexico locust, river willow.

CHARACTERISTIC ANIMALS:

Elk, beaver, bobcat, fox, Abert's squirrel.

NORTHERN CONIFEROUS FOREST

8,200 feet to 10,000 feet

Cool summer, cold winters high amounts of rain and snow, evaporation modest to low.

CHARACTERISTIC PLANTS:

Douglas fir, white fir, Englemann spruce, blue spruce, alpine juniper, limber pine, bristlecone pine, aspen.

CHARACTERISTIC ANIMALS:

High populations of elk, Rocky Mountain bighorn sheep, mountain marmot.

ALPINE TIMBERLINE AND ABOVE

10,000 feet and up (Timberline varies in elevation depending upon latitude and slope)

Temperatures cool to cold, high amounts of rain and snow, high evaporation, high wind, high exposure, severe weather possible any time of year.

CHARACTERISTIC PLANTS:

Low hardy grasses, dwarf shrubs and sedges, algae, lichens.

CHARACTERISTIC ANIMALS:

High populations of elk, Rocky Mountain bighorn sheep.

CAMPING ON NATIVE AMERICAN TRIBAL LANDS

NEW MEXICO OFFERS OUTDOOR RECREATIONAL opportunities such as camping, fishing, and hunting on Native American Tribal Land that some states do not provide. Many of these communities welcome campers. Most of the facilities are primitive, and many are not designed for RV camping, so pack up your tent and set your course.

Every Native American Nation has laws to preserve its own culture. Remember, you are visiting a sovereign nation within our nation. The rule of law is set by tribal council and enforced within its boundaries.

The land holds sacred religious significance to each tribe, and laws vary from nation to nation. Preservation of the tribal culture and heritage is a priority that runs deep within each nation. Remember, visiting here is a privilege.

The following are laws and observances that are typical to most Native American nations:

- **OBEY TRIBAL LAW ENFORCEMENT:** Federal, state, or county law enforcement have no jurisdiction on tribal lands.
- **VIOLATION OF TRAFFIC LAWS** may carry stiff penalties and fines, including mandatory appearance before a tribal magistrate.
- **PHOTOGRAPHY OR ARTISTIC RENDERING OF TRIBAL MEMBERS,** the land, or properties is, in most cases, strongly prohibited.
- **AUDIO RECORDING DEVICES** are, in most cases, strongly prohibited.
- **ALCOHOL POSSESSION AND/OR CONSUMPTION** on tribal property may be prohibited. Narcotic and/or drug possession and consumption is always strongly prohibited.
- **POSSESSION OF FIREARMS** without a tribal hunting license is prohibited.
- **RESERVATION FISHING AND HUNTING LICENSES** must be purchased from the specific tribal authority; New Mexico State fishing and hunting licenses are not valid.
- **SPECIFIC AREAS OF THE LAND MAY BE OFF LIMITS** to nontribal members for religious or sacred reasons. Please closely observe all signs and postings.
- **NATIVE AMERICAN CEMETERIES AND BURIAL GROUNDS ARE SACRED.** Do not enter unless invited.
- **MANY TRIBES CLOSE THE NATION'S LANDS FOR SPECIAL RELIGIOUS OBSERVANCES,** festivals, or tribal holidays. Check with the proper authority for sites that may be open to the public.
- **WHEN SPEAKING TO TRIBAL MEMBERS,** replace the term "Indian" with the words "Native American." Many tribes do not find the word "Indian" offensive; however, by using the term "Native American," tribal members understand you are conveying respect for their culture and the ethnic people as a whole.

- **NATIVE AMERICANS CONSIDER THEMSELVES AS A SEPARATE ETHNIC RACE,** and each tribe considers itself a unique community and culture. Most nations welcome visitors and depend on the sale of arts and crafts for their livelihood.

- **CERTAIN TRIBAL FESTIVALS ARE OPEN TO THE PUBLIC.** Do not ask questions unless encouraged to do so; instead, observe and learn. Tribal customs are not openly discussed with nontribal persons.

- **SPEAKING THE NAME OF DECEASED NATIVE AMERICANS,** such as Sitting Bull, Geronimo, Cochise or others, may be construed as disrespectful to the tribe, the ancestors, or the deceased individual.

- **PETS ARE ALLOWED AT CAMPGROUNDS UNDER FULL RESTRAINT,** but are not welcome in most other areas the tribal community. Most nations do not restrain their own dogs, and they are allowed to run freely. Please drive safely. Do not attempt to feed or pet these animals.

- **LIVESTOCK ROAM FREELY THROUGHOUT MOST TRIBAL LANDS.** Accidental injury to livestock may carry stiff penalties and fines, including appearance before a tribal magistrate and monetary compensation to the owner of the livestock.

- **DO NOT LITTER.** Littering is punishable in the tribal courts.

- **STAY ON MAIN ROADS** and state highways.

- **DO NOT REMOVE POTSHERDS,** feathers, arrowheads, stone tools, or other artifacts.

- **HARVESTING PLANTS,** berries, pinons, and medicinal plants may be prohibited.

- **HIKING, MOUNTAIN BIKING,** off-road motorcycle, or ATV riding may be prohibited.

T HE SCOUTING MOTTO IS "ALWAYS BE PREPARED." There is no reason to ever abort a camping trip if you plan well. Here are a few insights to help a tent camper enjoy outings.

LOW-IMPACT CAMPING

The old cliché "Take only photos; leave only footprints" is just plain common sense advice for campers. Years ago, people cut tree boughs for tent poles and under-tent bedding. Folks would trench around their tents, scarring the land. Those days are long gone, and we need to be wiser. Some campgrounds profiled in this book have a pack-it-in, pack-it-out policy. If someone leaves trash, do the right thing and pack it out. Think of the campsite you are renting as your home; it is! Public land belongs to you as well as all citizens!

KEEP A CLEAN CAMP

Not only does a clean camp discourage visits by varmints, but it is appreciated by the camper who comes after you. Leave your camp cleaner than you found it, always think of the next party who camps here. Cleaning up messes left by thoughtless campers is not the duty of the campground host. Make a habit of picking up even the smallest objects during the entire duration of your visit.

CAMPGROUND ETIQUETTE

It has been said, you can choose your friends, but you cannot choose your relatives or neighbors. The best way to maintain a peaceful campground is to be a good neighbor. Campers can be some of the friendliest folks you will ever cross paths with, and most live by the golden rule. Here are some good-neighbor policies we can all ascribe to:

- **COMPLY WITH ALL POSTED RULES.**
- **HOLD EVERYONE ACCOUNTABLE** in your party to comply with rules.
- **OBSERVE QUIET TIMES,** usually 10 p.m. to 8 a.m.
- **KEEP QUIET ENOUGH DURING DAYLIGHT HOURS** to hear the breezes in the trees.
- **NEVER POINT FLASHLIGHTS AT OTHERS** or into other campsites.
- **AVOID SETTING OFF VEHICLE ALARMS,** and gently shut vehicle doors..
- **BE FRIENDLY,** but have a light touch with others.
- **OFFER ASSISTANCE WHENEVER POSSIBLE** without being intrusive.
- **OFFER TO KEEP AN EYE ON YOUR NEIGHBOR'S CAMPSITE** if they are leaving; they will generally offer you the same security.
- **REPORT INAPPROPRIATE BEHAVIOR** to a campground host or a ranger. Don't take the law into your own hands.

- **NEVER ENTER ANOTHER PERSON'S CAMPSITE** without permission. Always walk around the campsite.

- **NEVER BORROW** from neighboring campers.

- **KEEP PETS QUIET** or leave them at home.

- **KEEP PETS ON A LEASH** and pick up after them.

- **WATCH YOUR CHILDREN CLOSELY;** teach them to have a light touch with strangers.

- **DRIVE SLOWLY IN CAMP** (5 to 10 miles per hour) and do not raise a dust.

- **IF YOU PLAY MUSIC,** use headphones.

- **RESPECT CAMPGROUND HOSTS** and rangers; they are there for your benefit.

FIRE SAFETY

It is mandatory to carry a shovel and axe (or hatchet) when you camp in New Mexico. When tent camping, carry a lawn rake as well, and rake a large radius free of combustibles from around the fire ring. Please use only water to douse your campfire, do not use dirt. Discard cold ashes in trash bags, not under trees or in streams.

WEATHER

The Land of Enchantment is known for enchanting weather! Due to its southerly location, New Mexico has a climate that attracts scores of outdoor enthusiasts. Springtime comes earlier than it does for our neighbors to the north, and fall remains longer. For the "fair weather" outdoors enthusiast, this means the camping season can begin as early as March and can extend well into November. Many campgrounds open as early as March to accommodate spring turkey hunts and remain open late for elk and deer hunting. Many campers begin their treks in early spring in the lowland desert, moving to the higher elevations as the weather warms, then return to the lower elevations in late fall.

Spring is the most variable season. During March you'll find your first signs of rebirth in the lowlands, yet trees in the high country reach full foliage by late May to early June. Both winter- and summerlike weather can occur in spring. New Mexico is notoriously windy in the spring and the fall, so be prepared.

Through mid-May, the high country can experience daytime temperatures of 60°F and nighttime temperatures that drop below freezing. Be prepared for cold fronts—temperatures can rapidly drop, and cold-weather apparel is not optional. Keep an eye on the forecast, pack warm sleeping bags, and have cold-weather apparel handy. New Mexico's spring weather is usually dry, and stage ll fire restrictions (no campfires allowed) are common.

Desert campgrounds in the lowlands are ideal locations to begin the camping season, with daytime temperatures in the 60°F-to-70°F range and nighttime temperatures in the 40°F-to-50°F range. This is the ideal time to experience the Chihuahuan Desert. Many southern New Mexico campgrounds have cacti and succulent gardens, which begin blooming in March and continue to do so through the month of May. Desert yucca blooms at the same time, with incredible white blossoms bending in the warm breezes. Sage begins growing at the same time, painting the desert floors a silvery green.

Summers begin in mid-May in the high country. June temperatures can soar into the

80°F range but rarely go higher. Nights are usually cool and can drop into the mid-40s at night at elevations of 8,000 feet or more. As July approaches, the "monsoon season" arrives, dousing the thirsty mountains with much-needed rain. The rains bring cold fronts, and temperatures that plummet into the 40°F-to-50°F range are common. Precipitation levels have increased significantly since 2005, bringing rain on an almost daily basis to many areas, so pack that rain gear and have a tarp handy for the picnic table.

Lowland-desert camping in summer can be challenging, and temperatures in excess of 100°F are common. The lakes and rivers throughout the state are popular and become quite crowded. Sunscreen and polarized sunglasses are essential; the New Mexico sun is bright. Sunstroke is a constant danger, so take precautions and stay hydrated. Shade is a priority, but campgrounds with adequate shade trees are uncommon in the desert, so a shade shelter is a wise investment.

Our desert campgrounds are delightful when the "monsoon season" arrives—hiking in the warm summer rain is a wonderful experience. Summer sunrises and sunsets are incredible, with clouds on the horizon; majestic pinks fiery reds and yellows paint New Mexico skies with indescribable beauty.

Autumn arrives in the high country in mid-September, and most campgrounds close by October, with the exception of campgrounds near popular hunting areas. U.S. Forest Service campgrounds may lock some loops because of dwindling crowds. Fall usually sees an increase of activity in the lowlands, with the warm autumn days hovering around 70°F to 80°F until November. Evening temperatures in the lowlands rarely drop below 40°F through November.

The first snows of winter usually arrive in the higher elevations in November, and snow can continue through April. Annual winter snowfall can vary from 40 to 120 inches. Expect to incur entire days of below-freezing weather; temperatures may range from mild to bitterly cold. High-country campgrounds usually close at the first signs of snow and usually open after the snow has melted. A few state-park campgrounds will remain open. Always call ahead for campground-closure information.

The lowland-desert campgrounds in the southern parts of New Mexico become quite busy in the winter. Snowbirds arrive in November and stay until March, fueling the economies of many communities with much-needed revenue. Winter tent camping is delightful in the deserts, with daytime temperatures in the 50°F-to-60°F range and nights in the 30°F-to-40°F range.

VARMINTS

Most campgrounds profiled in this book will put you smack dab into bear country. In New Mexico we only have to deal with black bears; they can be a handful, and have killed people in New Mexico. Bears are able to smell food from a distance of up to 10 miles. Bears and other varmints remember and return to campsites where the opportunity for a meal is at it's best.

Keep your food inaccessible, don't cook close to the tent, and make sure your potty is at least 200 feet from the tent site. Always change the clothes you cook in before you head for the sleeping bag.

Most varmint's sense of smell is about 500 times more sensitive than a human, so do not store any food or the clothing you cooked in inside your tent. Always dispose of trash before bedtime. Some campsites require you to pack out what you pack in. Remember while in bear country, cologne, aftershave, and scented deodorants attract bears.

Keep your pets on a leash and under control at all times. Coyote and fox generally don't frequent campgrounds, but they are shrewd predators and will snatch unattended pets. Mountain lion and bobcat are rarely sighted, but be wary. Utilizing bear proofing methods will help ensure that varmints will not be attracted to your camp. Mexican wolves were controversially re-introduced in the Gila Mountains in the 1990s; they are successfully breeding in the Gila.

Rodents can get into food, so keep everything packed away when you aren't cooking. Raccoons can wreak havoc at your campground. Haunta Virus, plague, and other diseases are carried by campground rodents.

New Mexico has rattlesnakes; do your homework, and be wary especially with children and pets. Carry a snake-bite kit and know how to properly use it. Teach children how to avoid potential snake encounters.

By all means, keep your tent zipped shut at all times when camping in New Mexico. Mosquitoes aren't quite as common as in many other states due to the arid climate. Bees and wasps are most common around rivers and lakes. Be prepared for encounters with snakes, scorpions, and centipedes. Don't leave your footwear outside of the tent, and make a habit of shaking out your shoes and boots prior to putting them on.

BLACK BEARS

New Mexico has one species of bear, the North American Black Bear (*Ursus americanus*). Black bears are not an endangered species, and it is estimated that up to 5,000 bears reside in New Mexico with a population of over 900,000 in North America. Campgrounds at more than 5,000 feet elevation in New Mexico are in bear country.

Since 2000, 14 deaths have been linked to black-bear attacks. There have been 56 documented human deaths by black bears in North America in the past 100 years. Black bears generally attack humans only when provoked or startled. In August 2001, an elderly lady was attacked and killed by a black bear at her home near Mora, New Mexico. In 2007, a 12-year-old boy was bitten in the hand at night while swatting at a bear who was sniffing around his tent at Sugarite Canyon State Park, near Raton, New Mexico. The campground host at Southfork Campground near Bonito Lake reported that a bear damaged numerous items around his trailer in the spring of 2007. The campground host at Jemez Falls Campground had a two-week period in the summer of 2007 where four different bears invaded the campground. There have been many other reported confrontations with bears in New Mexico.

FAST FACTS ABOUT BLACK BEARS

- **BLACK BEARS ARE THE MOST COMMON SPECIES** of bear in North America.
- **ADULT MALE BEARS WEIGH UP TO 600 POUNDS,** female bears weigh up to 400 pounds.

- **STANDING UP ON ITS HIND FEET,** a black bear can tower up to seven feet tall.
- **THOUGH BLACK BEARS GENERALLY HAVE SHAGGY BLACK HAIR,** the coat can vary in color from white to chocolate-brown, cinnamon-brown, and blonde. They occasionally have a slight V-shaped white chest blaze.
- **BLACK BEARS HAVE A LARGE RANGE** that can encompass hundreds of square miles.
- **BLACK BEARS CAN RUN OVER 30 MILES PER HOUR,** are adept at climbing trees, and are excellent swimmers.
- **BLACK BEARS RARELY MAKE FALSE CHARGES** to intimidate; if the bear lunges, it will attack.
- **BLACK BEARS HUNT AND FORAGE** mostly at night, and are less active during the day.
- **BLACK BEARS SEE IN COLOR** and their vision is equal to that of a human; night vision is far superior.
- **BLACK BEARS' HEARING EXCEEDS HUMAN FREQUENCY RANGES** and is estimated at twice the sensitivity.
- **BLACK BEARS HAVE A KEEN SENSE OF SMELL,** estimated at 500 times the sensitivity of a human. Bears have an ability to detect food up to a distance of 10 miles.
- **BLACK BEARS CAN LIVE UP TO 33 YEARS.**

BEAR-PROOFING YOUR CAMP

- **CONSULT WITH RANGERS,** camp hosts, and other campers regarding recent bear sightings.
- **ABIDE BY ALL POSTED WARNING SIGNS** and bulletins posted by the ranger office.
- **KEEP ALL FOOD STORED** in vehicle or animal-proof storage lockers between meals, and when leaving the campsite, even for short periods of time.
- **STOW COOKWARE,** all spices, and hummingbird feeders while away from camp, and overnight inside a vehicle or animal-proof storage lockers.
- **KEEP A CLEAN CAMP;** throw trash away frequently.
- **NEVER THROW ANY FOOD ITEMS** in the campfire.
- **NEVER TAKE ANY FOODS** or drinks inside tents.
- **STORE ANY CLOTHING** that was worn while preparing food or eating a meal inside of a vehicle.
- **KEEP PETS ON LEASHES** at all times. Pets are a very good early warning alarm when bears are near.
- **DISPOSE OF UNFINISHED BEER** and sugary drinks away from your camp.

IF A BEAR ENTERS YOUR CAMP

- **DO NOT PANIC** and do not run; gather all members of your party and your pets, and quietly get in your vehicle, or lock yourself in the toilet building if you have to.
- **KEEP CAR DOORS UNLOCKED** during the day while in camp for quick entry.
- **MAKE EVERY ATTEMPT TO AVOID** confronting the bear if possible. Use bear repellent only, do not use pepper spray meant for humans or dogs.
- **USE WHISTLES OR CAR PANIC ALARMS** in an attempt to scare the bear away.

- **AS A LAST RESORT, KILL AN ATTACKING BEAR;** use a weapon of no less than .38 caliber. A warning shot may not stop a charge.

POISONOUS SNAKES

FAST FACTS ABOUT POISONOUS SNAKES

All venomous snakes in New Mexico are very dangerous and all should be avoided at all costs. Snakes can be upset by human presence and can unexpectedly become aggressive. Do not give them a reason or an opportunity to attack. Always keep your distance. Your safety is your responsibility.

Familiarize yourself with the snakes of the area you are traveling into, both venomous and nonvenomous species. Reptile guidebooks are beneficial for identification, but the best way to prevent a snakebite is to steer clear of all species of snake. Learn which habitats the venomous species in your region are likely to be encountered in, and use caution when in those habitats. Always take a buddy into the field with you; do not hike alone. Wear ankle-high boots and loose-fitting pants.

Do not take a snake by surprise; make noise on the trail. Stay on trails, and watch where you place your hands and feet, especially when climbing or stepping over fences, large rocks, and logs, or when collecting firewood. At the campground, tread cautiously around rock outcroppings and downed trees.

Of the 8,000 snakebite victims in the United States each year, only about 10 to 15 die. However, for any snakebite, the best course of action is to get medical care as soon as possible.

- **KEEP THE SNAKEBITE VICTIM STILL,** as movement helps the venom spread through the body.

- **KEEP THE INJURED BODY PART MOTIONLESS** and just below heart level.

- **KEEP THE VICTIM WARM,** calm, and at rest, and transport the victim immediately to medical care. Do not allow victim to eat or drink anything.

- **IF MEDICAL CARE IS MORE THAN HALF AN HOUR AWAY,** wrap a bandage a few inches above the bite, keeping it loose enough to enable blood flow (you should be able to fit a finger beneath it). Do not cut off blood flow with a tight tourniquet. Leave the bandage in place until reaching medical care.

- **IF YOU HAVE A SNAKEBITE KIT,** wash the bite, and place the kit's suction device over the bite. (Do not suck the poison out with your mouth.) Do not remove the suction device until you reach a medical facility.

- **TRY TO IDENTIFY THE SNAKE** so that the proper antivenin can be administered, but do not waste time or endanger yourself trying to capture or kill it.

- **IF YOU ARE ALONE AND ON FOOT,** start walking slowly toward help, exerting the injured area as little as possible. If you run or if the bite has delivered a large amount of venom, you may collapse, but a snakebite seldom results in death.

The five most common venomous snakes in New Mexico are the timber rattlesnake, diamondback rattlesnake, sidewinder rattlesnake, speckled rattlesnake, and western coral snake. The four rattlesnake species belong to the pit-viper family, and the coral snake belongs to the cobra family. The fangs of the cobra-snake family are fixed in place, and do not fold back inside the lower jaw as do pit-viper fangs.

TIMBER RATTLESNAKE (*CROTALUS HORRIDUS*) 35–74"

Colors of snake range from yellowish-, brownish- or pinkish-gray, with tan or reddish-brown back stripe dividing chevronlike cross bands. There are dark stripes behind the eyes. Timber rattlesnakes are active from April to October; in the daytime in spring and fall, at night in summer. Timber rattlesnakes congregate in large numbers about rocky den sites. They are often encountered coiled up waiting for prey (squirrel, mice, chipmunks, small birds); if you see one, remain motionless. Record longevity exceeds 30 years. Timber rattlesnakes make their abode in elevations of more than 6,600 feet and are the most common rattlesnake species found in the high elevations of New Mexico.

WESTERN DIAMONDBACK RATTLESNAKE (*CROTALUS ATROX*) 34–83"

This is the largest Western rattlesnake. The snake is heavy bodied with large head sharply distinct from neck. The back is patterned with light-bordered dark diamonds or hexagonal blotches. There are two light diagonal lines on each side of its face. A stripe behind the eye meets the upper lip well in front of the angle of the jaw. The snake's tail is encircled by broad black-and-white rings. Known as the "coon tail rattler," this dangerous reptile is most active late in the day and at night during hot summer months, but can been seen from April through October. It eats rodents and birds. Record longevity is nearly 26 years. When disturbed it stands its ground, lifts its head well above its coils, and sounds a buzzing warning. Its habitat is in arid and semiarid areas from plains to mountains: brushy desert, rocky canyons, bluffs along rivers, sparsely vegetated rocky foothills; sea level to 7,000 feet.

SIDEWINDER (*CROTALUS CERASTES*) 17–32"

The sidewinder is a rough-scaled rattler with a prominent triangular, hornlike projection over each eye. It travels over surfaces by "sidewinding." It leaves a trail of parallel J-shaped markings behind it. Primarily nocturnal, it is usually encountered crossing roads between sundown and midnight in spring. During the day it occupies mammal burrows or hides in shelters beneath bushes. The sidewinder eats pocket mice, kangaroo rats, and lizards. This snake is active from April to October, and active late in the day and at night during hot summer months. This snake predominately prefers arid desert flatland and sandy arroyos, and is found up to 5,000 feet of elevation.

SPECKLED RATTLESNAKE (*CROTALUS MITCHELLII*) 23–52"

This rattlesnake's pattern and color vary greatly; it is most commonly seen with a sandy, speckled appearance. The rattlesnake is active during the day in spring and fall, at night in summer. It eats ground squirrel, kangaroo rats, white-footed mice, birds, and lizards. Record longevity exceeds 16 years. The rattlensnake prefers rugged rocky terrain, rock outcrops, deep canyons, talus, chaparral amid rock piles and boulders, and rocky foothills up to 8,000 feet in elevation.

WESTERN CORAL SNAKE (*MICRUROIDES EURYXANTHUS*) 13–21"

The western coral snake is blunt-snouted and glossy, with alternating wide red, wide black, and narrow yellow or white rings encircling the body. The head is uniformly black to the angle of the jaw; its scales are smooth. This snake emerges at night, usually during or following a warm shower. When disturbed, it buries its head in its coils, raises and exposes the underside of its tail, and may make a popping sound. This snake is the most dangerous snake in New Mexico, and its venom is highly toxic. The western coral snake eats blind snakes or other small snakes. It prefers rocky areas, plains to lower mountain slopes, rocky upland desert—especially in arroyos and river bottoms up to 5,900 feet in elevation.

SCORPIONS AND CENTIPEDES

Scorpions have long been of interest to humans primarily because of their ability to give painful and sometimes life-threatening stings. Scorpions are venomous arthropods in the class *Arachnida,* relatives of spiders, mites, ticks, and others. Scorpions have an elongated body and a segmented tail that is tipped with a venomous stinger. They have four pairs of legs and plierlike pincers, which are used for grasping. The species include:

THE DESERT GRASSLAND SCORPION (*PARUROCTONUS UTAHENSIS*)

The desert grassland scorpion spends most of its reclusive life in its burrow to minimize exposure to predation. The venom of this scorpion results in a painful sting, but its rarely fatal unless an allergic reaction occurs. This species of scorpion resides in shifting sands in the Mexican state of Chihuahua, and in Arizona, New Mexico, Texas, and Utah. This scorpion is pale yellow to yellowish-brown matching local sand color. Pincers are swollen and keeled with short fingers in adults. Legs have bristle combs that provide traction on sandy ground. An obligate burrower, it often digs its burrow at the base of vegetation on sand dunes. This species potentially lives six to seven years.

DESERT HAIRY SCORPION (*HADRURUS ARIZONENSIS*)

The desert hairy scorpion is the largest scorpion in North America, obtaining a length up to six inches. Their bodies are brown, with yellowish pinchers and legs. Their common name comes from the brown hairs that cover their bodies. It is not a dangerous scorpion to humans unless an allergic reaction occurs. This species is aggressive, though, and will sting readily. The desert hairy scorpion gets its water from the animals it feeds on. This has proven to be a popular scorpion species in captivity due to its size, beauty, and low risk of danger.

ARIZONA BARK SCORPION (*CENTRUROIDES SCULPTURATUS*)

This species is universally tan and grows to a length of two-and-a-half inches; it is the most commonly encountered house scorpion. The Arizona bark scorpion is the only species in North America with venom potent enough to be dangerous to humans. The sting of this scorpion can be fatal to humans, particularly to infants and small children, so it is important to be careful when picking up firewood or rocks. Although the sting of this scorpion has killed more people in Arizona than all types of poisonous snakes combined, not one documented death has occurred in the United States for more than 30 years.

GIANT REDHEADED CENTIPEDE (*SCOLOPENDRA HEROS GIRARD*)

Centipedes, named for the erroneous belief that they have 100 feet, rarely have more than 60 or 70 feet. These centipedes attract a great deal of attention because of their fierce appearance and size, growing up to eight inches long.

The centipede's bite is followed by a sharp and strictly local pain which subsides after about 15 minutes. In about two hours the pain is only very slight, but there is a general swelling in the bite location. Three hours after the bite, most symptoms will disappear. The bite of a typical centipede can be very painful for humans, similar to that of a wasp sting, and can usually be treated with an antihistamine if no infection develops. Centipede bites to children and those who are allergic will require prompt medical attention.

After dealing with the subjects of snakes, scorpions, and centipedes, there should be no doubt as to why it is wise to keep tents zipped completely!

MAPS

The old saying "plan your work, then work your plan" is good advice for campers. The U.S. Forest Service and Bureau of Land Management offices sell topographical maps.

Topographical software is an excellent resource because you can print your maps. I used both DeLorme Topo USA and National Geographic Topo! for researching this book. I love the *New Mexico Road and Recreation Atlas,* published by Benchmark Maps.

GPS is new, reliable technology, and it is an intelligent investment for the camper. It is wise to carry a compass and trail map when hiking. Always let someone know when you leave and give them an expected time of your return. Always register at trailheads or forest service offices.

FOUR-WHEEL DRIVE

All back-country campgrounds profiled in this book can be reached under normal road conditions without four-wheel drive; most SUVs or pickup trucks with reasonable ground clearance will get you to all of these campgrounds just fine. Road conditions will be described if risky conditions exist. Road conditions can change rapidly. The smooth dirt road I describe can become mud-bogged and impassable in a matter of minutes in a flash flood. Intelligently calculate, and call ahead for road conditions. Do not take unnecessary risks.

WATER POTABILITY

If you decide to bring water jugs to fill at the campground, there are precautions you should take to ensure water purity. I use the TastePURE brand water filter from Camco Manufacturing. It is an inline filter for RVs and lasts tent campers several years. Every campground treats well water with chlorine to kill bacteria, which may be noticeable in the smell and taste. Therefore, filtering is universally recommended.

COMFORT

Camping in New Mexico, you will find nice grassy forest floors are the exception rather than the rule. Rocky soil and hard-packed caliche clay are common. When investing in a good ground pad, shop for quality. The best ground pads are self-inflating, with adequate foam padding inside.

Avoid using inflatable air mattresses; New Mexico has cornered the market on its variety of thorns and stickers. Murphy's Law states: thorns attached to clothing will systematically puncture air mattresses no matter how careful you are. In colder weather, air mattresses have poor insulating quality.

GEAR BOX

See Appendix A for the camping-equipment checklist.

NORTH CENTRAL CAMPGROUNDS:
Carson National Forest

01
CANJILON LAKES
CAMPGROUNDS

CANJILON (PRONOUNCED CAN—HEE—LOAN) Lakes is a beautiful remote campground. Located several miles west of the tiny community of Canjilon, along bumpy Forest Service 129. Automobiles can make the trip driving slowly, but four-wheel-drive vehicles are recommended. Some areas on the road will slow you to 5 to 10 miles per hour. I towed a small pop-up here years ago, and will never do it again.

The washboard road is a reason why most RVs aren't as willing to make the trip, so this makes these two campgrounds an ideal tent-camper's retreat. Even so, there will be a few hearty RVs that tread the road.

Three cold-water lakes are located just 3 miles apart, Lower Canjilon Lake Campground has 11 sites, and Middle Canjilon Lake Campground has 32 sites. Upper Canjilon Lake has no campground but has several picnic tables and a vault toilet for picnics and fishing. Area fishing is excellent, primarily for rainbow, brook, and cutthroat trout. (It should be mentioned that there are two other campgrounds in the area, Canjilon Creek, with 4 campsites, and Trout Lakes, with 11 campsites. The latter is accessible only by four-wheel-drive vehicles; neither are profiled in this book.)

The altitude here is among the highest of all of the campgrounds profiled in this book. It dips down to the 40°F range most nights; even in July. Daytime temperatures rarely exceed 80°F. It can snow here anytime during the camping season. Road conditions may deteriorate during the New Mexico monsoon season, from early July all the way through September. The campgrounds are open from Memorial Day through Labor Day.

The altitude is partly what makes Canjilon so lovely. There are many aspen groves, tall ponderosa

> *Meadows of wildflowers abound, including Indian paintbrush and columbine.*

RATINGS

Beauty: ✿ ✿ ✿ ✿ ✿
Privacy: ✿ ✿ ✿ ✿
Spaciousness: ✿ ✿ ✿ ✿ ✿
Quiet: ✿ ✿ ✿ ✿ ✿
Security: ✿ ✿ ✿ ✿
Cleanliness: ✿ ✿ ✿ ✿ ✿

KEY INFORMATION

ADDRESS: Canjilon Ranger District
P.O. Box 488
Canjilon, NM 87515
(505) 684-2486
www.fs.fed.us/r3/carson

OPERATED BY: Canjilon Ranger District
Carson National Forest
U.S. Department of Agriculture

OPEN: Official season, Memorial Day–Labor Day

SITES: 41 individual sites; all sites are first come, first served; 11 sites in Lower Canjilon Lakes Campground; 30 sites in Middle Cajilon Lakes Campground

EACH SITE HAS: Parking space, picnic table, and fire ring

REGISTRATION: Self-service registration, immediately upon selecting campsite

FEE: $10 per night

ELEVATION: Lower Campground 9,850 feet; Middle Campground: 9,830 feet

RESTRICTIONS: *Pets:* On leash, 6-foot maximum; take precautionary measures for predators
Fires: Wood fires permitted in fire rings; charcoal grills are permitted
Alcohol: Within campsite only
Quiet Hours: 10 p.m.–8 a.m.
Stay Limit: 14 days

pines, spruce, and fir. There is scrub oak near the lakes and creeks. You will see many wildflowers abounding, including Indian paintbrush and columbine. Outside the campgrounds are open meadows with tall prairie grass waving in the cool mountain breezes.

You will see some aspen groves defoliated in this area. These trees died as a result of an infestation of western tent caterpillars, with past drought conditions contributing to their demise. Western tent caterpillars are widespread throughout the forests of the southwest, 35,800 acres fell victim in New Mexico alone.

Several hiking trails exist nearby, which will tire you quickly due to the altitude. Nearby Canjilon Mountain tops out at 10,913 feet. Red Hill just due west is 10,108 feet at its summit. This entire area is more than 9,000 feet in elevation.

Most campsites are shady through the day and vary in size and privacy. Select your campsite with regard to water runoff, because some locations become a mud bog. Many of the sites are grassy and are ideal for tent camping. These two campgrounds rarely fill to capacity.

Each campsite comes with a fire ring and a picnic table. The vault toilets are modern and very clean. There is no evidence of vandalism, and Forest Service law enforcement officers patrol frequently, with an occasional visit by New Mexico Department of Game and Fish, and the Rio Arriba County Sheriff's Department. The security of these campgrounds is great. Fishing licenses and possession limits are checked here on a regular basis, so beware.

There is no water here, but you can fill at the Canjilon Ranger Station on the way up. Filtering the water is recommended. The Ranger Station is 1 mile north of the town of Canjilon on FR 129. Be sure to come well supplied, because the bumpy drive to town isn't something you want to do once you get settled in.

This is black bear country; watch for mountain lion, bobcat, and coyote as well. You will see evidence of beaver along nearby Canjilon Creek. Raccoons are regular pests here as well. There are no bear-proof food lockers, so store all food items in your vehicle.

MAP

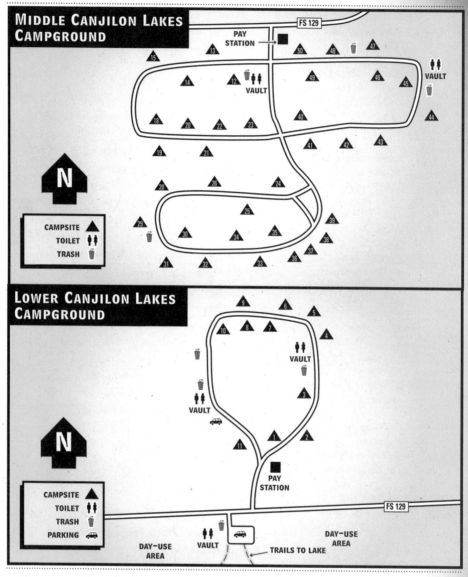

MIDDLE CANJILON LAKES CAMPGROUND

FS 129

PAY STATION

CAMPSITE ▲
TOILET
TRASH

VAULT

VAULT

LOWER CANJILON LAKES CAMPGROUND

VAULT

VAULT

PAY STATION

CAMPSITE ▲
TOILET
TRASH
PARKING

FS 129

DAY-USE AREA

VAULT

TRAILS TO LAKE

DAY-USE AREA

GPS COORDINATES

LOWER LAKES
UTM Zone (WGS84) 13S
Easting 0379632
Northing 4045844
Latitude N 36° 33' 0.2"
Longtitude W 106° 20' 41.6"

MIDDLE LAKES
UTM Zone (WGS84) 13S
Easting 0380755
Northing 4046386
Latitude N 36° 33' 19.7"
Longtitude W 106° 19' 56.8"

GETTING THERE

From the town of Canjilon, Drive northeast on FS 129 and Lower Canjilon Lake is 12 miles, on the left side of the road. Middle Canjilon Lake is 1 mile farther.

02
CHACO CANYON
CAMPGROUND

> *You can hear the spirits of the old ones haunting the canyons.*

HOW WOULD YOU LIKE TO CAMP within a few steps from ancient Anasazi cliff dwellings? If so, Chaco is the place. Some say you can hear strange sounds at night, the spirits of the old ones haunting the canyons. I heard no spirits, just the rain spattering my tent until way past midnight. I spent the evening reading all I could of the Anasazi culture that placed its indelible marks upon this beautiful canyon desert land.

The Navajo, Hopi, and most New Mexico Pueblo Indian cultures hold this land sacred, so please be respectful and observe posted signs. The area is used by many tribes for religious ceremonies at different times of the year.

Chaco Canyon was a major Pueblo cultural center from AD 850 until 1250. Known for architecture, astronomy, and artistry, the visitor center has a museum with beautiful pottery displays and informative insight into the Anasazi way of life. A well-stocked bookstore with souvenirs supports the museum. A domed observatory for viewing the starry skies over Chaco Canyon is free. Please inquire at the visitor center for operating times. Visitors are encouraged to bring their own telescopes. Several times a year different astronomy groups come to celebrate the incredible night skies with "star parties."

Past the visitor center are five ruins along a 9-mile circular loop, open from daybreak to dusk. The rock work of the ruins is amazing, and the engineering and construction skills of the Anasazi are the real attraction at this location.

Mountain biking is allowed on certain trails with a free permit. Hiking the ruins is easy, but bring your camera, sunscreen, hat, and water. Between the Pueblo Bonito ruins and the Chetro Ketl ruins is an amazing petroglyph trail, preserving 13 sites where pictographs

RATINGS

Beauty: ✿ ✿ ✿
Privacy: ✿ ✿ ✿
Spaciousness: ✿ ✿ ✿
Quiet: ✿ ✿ ✿
Security: ✿ ✿ ✿ ✿ ✿
Cleanliness: ✿ ✿ ✿ ✿ ✿

can be seen and photographed. Interpretive booklets are available along the trail for a donation of 50 cents.

The campground is located off the right side of the paved access road one-half mile east of the visitor center. This is not a pretty campground. The ground is sandy; desert sage, tumbleweeds, and wild grasses intermingle with a few desert wildflowers. The beauty comes in the evening, when the pink and orange sunset paints the canyon walls and mesas with indescribable colors. The warm evening breezes cool many a weary hiker, and the coyote's song can be heard for miles. Several night birds provide melodies, and owls can be heard throughout the night.

Due to a renovation of the campground's septic system, the 2007 camping season was extremely limited and only 30 sites of the 49 sites were open. Two modern restrooms are equipped with flushing toilets and sinks. Potable water is available at the visitor center, one-half mile away. After filtering the water still tasted funny but made incredible cowboy coffee. Bringing in potable water is recommended.

Each campsite is equipped with a picnic table, gravel tent box, and fire ring. All sites are level. Most campsites are fully exposed with no shade whatsoever. It is wise to bring a

KEY INFORMATION

ADDRESS:	Chaco Culture National Historical Park P.O. Box 220 Nageezi, NM 87037 505) 346-3900 www.nps.gov/chcu
OPERATED BY:	National Park Service U.S. Department of the Interior
OPEN:	Year-round; park is open 365 days a year; visitor center is open every day except Thanksgiving, Christmas Day, and New Year's Day in observance of these holidays, but the park's roads, sites, trails, and campground will remain open. The park is open every day from sunrise to sunset. The visitor center is open 8 a.m.–5 p.m.
SITES:	49 individual sites; all sites are first come, first served
EACH SITE HAS:	Parking space, picnic table, graveled tent box, and fire ring
REGISTRATION:	Park admission per vehicle is $8 and covers all occupants
FEE:	$10 per night single unit; register to camp at the visitor center
ELEVATION:	6,214 feet
RESTRICTIONS:	*Pets:* On leash, 6-foot long maximum; pets are not allowed on trails, or at ruins *Fires:* Wood fires permitted only in provided fire rings; charcoal grills are permitted *Alcohol:* Within campsite only *Quiet Hours:* 8 p.m.–8 a.m. *Stay Limit:* 14 days

MAP

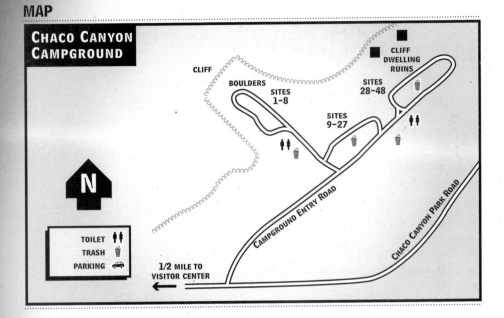

CHACO CANYON CAMPGROUND

CLIFF

BOULDERS

SITES 1-8

SITES 9-27

CLIFF DWELLING RUINS

SITES 28-48

N

TOILET
TRASH
PARKING

1/2 MILE TO VISITOR CENTER

CAMPGROUND ENTRY ROAD

CHACO CANYON PARK ROAD

GETTING THERE

Turn South off US 550 at CR 7900. This route is clearly signed from US 550 to the park boundary (21 miles). The route includes 8 miles of paved road (CR 7900) and 13 miles of rough dirt road (CR 7950).

GPS COORDINATES

UTM Zone (WGS84) 13S
Easting 0239140
Northing 3991414
Latitude 36 01'56.4"
Longtitude 107 53'42.5"

sun shelter, and sunscreen is not an option. Only two campsites are shaded by trees, and a few sites are scattered among the boulders, which afford a little more shade and good privacy. These boulders are habitat for various species of snakes, among them the prairie rattlesnake.

Like most desert canyon campgrounds, Chaco Canyon is best enjoyed in the spring and fall when the weather is cooler. At this latitude and altitude, snows frequently blanket the area in winter, so come prepared.

From US 550, you will travel a 22-mile road, mostly dirt but muddy in spots. You have to cross an arroyo, which can flood with little warning; heed the signs. If the current is swift, do not tempt fate.

Bring everything you need, because the 44-mile round-trip to US 550 takes you to a convenience store called the Forty-Four Store with very few supplies, and the town of Nageezi a few miles to the north has a trading post with limited groceries. Bring firewood because there is no firewood to gather inside the park.

JICARILLA APACHE LAKE CAMPGROUNDS

THE CROWN JEWEL OF NEW MEXICO'S Native American Tribal Lands is the Jicarilla Apache Nation. The Jicarilla lands are located in the scenic mountains and rugged mesas of northern New Mexico near the Colorado border. The Jicarilla lands are composed of nearly one million acres.

South of the town of Dulce, fishing abounds at five beautiful mountain lakes, from 30 to 400 acres in size. The lakes harbor thousands of ducks and the greatest variety of waterfowl found in the Southwest. Three lakes are set aside for camping.

The town of Dulce is the headquarters of the Jicarilla nation, and has two gas stations, several churches, and a modern grocery store. There are several gift shops selling arts and crafts, including the intricately woven baskets that the Jicarilla are famous for; in fact, the Spanish name *Jicarilla* means "little baskets."

Jicarilla Lake camping is primitive, and Enbom and Mundo lakes are inaccessible to RVs. Excellent beach camping is available at Stone Lake, but you will see RVs here occasionally. There is no water at any of the campgrounds; you can fill your water in Dulce, and filtering is recommended.

ENBOM LAKE

Enbom is the smallest of the lake campgrounds and offers only four campsites. Camping is free, but at least one member of each camping party must have a valid Jicarilla fishing permit. There are two campsites with picnic tables and a fire ring, and two sites with only a fire ring. The camp area is equipped with one portable toilet.

Some shade is on the north side of the lake provided by ponderosa pines. On the west side of the lake, two small peninsulas are ideal locations to set up camp, right along the shoreline. A fire ring is provided

> *The crown jewel of New Mexico's Native American Tribal Lands*

RATINGS

Beauty: ✪ ✪ ✪ ✪
Privacy: ✪ ✪ ✪
Spaciousness: ✪ ✪ ✪
Quiet: ✪ ✪
Security: ✪
Cleanliness: ✪ ✪ ✪

ADDRESS: Jicarilla Apache
Department of
Game and Fish
P.O. Box 313
Dulce, NM 87528
(505) 759-3255
www.jicarillahunt
.com/camping.php

OPERATED BY: Jicarilla Apache
Department of
Game and Fish,
Jicarilla Apache
Nation

OPEN: Official season,
Memorial Day–
Labor Day

SITES: Enbom Lake, 4;
Mundo Lake, 7;
Stone Lake, large
tenting area

EACH SITE HAS: Parking space,
picnic table, and
fire ring

REGISTRATION: Self-service
registration,
immediately upon
selecting campsite at
Mundo and Stone
Lake; no camping
fee at Embom Lake

FEE: Enbom Lake, free;
Mundo Lake, $5 per
night; Stone Lake,
$10 per night

RESTRICTIONS: *Pets:* On leash, 6-foot
maximum; take
precautionary
measures for
predators
Fires: Wood fires
permitted only in
provided fire rings;
charcoal grills are
permitted
Alcohol: Within
campsite only;
permitted but be
discreet
Quiet Hours: 10 p.m.–
8 a.m.
Stay Limit: 14 days

at each of these sites. No shade exists at these two locations. On the southwest corner of the lake, two other campsites are shaded by ponderosa pine. All sites offer privacy and are spacious.

Very little security exists at these facilities, but Jicarilla Game and Fish Department may patrol on occasion. There will be some road noise. The campground is close to the road, but traffic is light. All roads into this lake area are dirt, and can become impassable when wet.

MUNDO LAKE

Mundo Lake is twice as large as Enbom and has seven campsites available. Camping is $5 per night. The campsites are on the hill just north of the lake. These sites will be quite dusty; the ground is dirt, not grass. Several sites overlook the lake, but these sites are small and the ground is not level. There are seven fire rings and picnic tables and three shelters.

The camp area is equipped with one portable toilet. Fishing at these lakes is excellent, regular stocking and natural reproduction gives fishermen opportunities to land some pretty big fish. Stocked mostly with rainbow trout, the Jicarilla nation works closely with New Mexico Game and Fish, who provide restocking.

STONE LAKE

Stone Lake has a variety of camping options along its 3 miles of shoreline. Unfortunately there are no areas set aside specifically for tent camping. There are shelters, picnic tables, and fire rings at most sites. Tents and RVs are welcome at all of these sites. There is a 24-unit RV park located immediately southwest of Stone Lake on Road J-8.

This graveled park has electricity, water, and sewer hookups for RV's and camp trailers, with a spectacular view of Stone Lake and Horse Lake Mesa. $10 camping fee per night is made at a self-service unit, located at the park entrance. At least one member of each camping party must have a valid Jicarilla fishing permit.

MAP

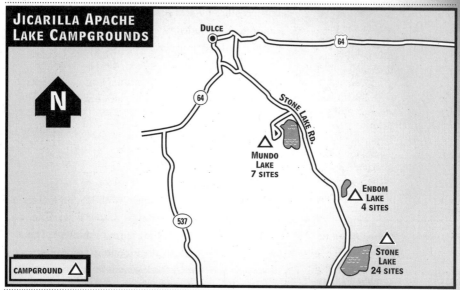

JICARILLA APACHE LAKE CAMPGROUNDS

DULCE

64

N

STONE LAKE RD.

△ MUNDO LAKE 7 SITES

△ ENBOM LAKE 4 SITES

64

537

△ STONE LAKE 24 SITES

CAMPGROUND △

GETTING THERE

To get to Enbom Lake: from Dulce, take Stone Lake Road (J-8), 12 miles southeast to Enbom Lake. Turn off to left.

To get to Mundo Lake: from Dulce, take Stone Lake Road (J-8), 6 miles southeast to Mundo Lake. Turn off to right.

To get to Stone Lake: from Dulce, take Stone Lake Road (J-8), 17 miles southeast to Stone Lake. Turn off to left.

GPS COORDINATES

ENBOM LAKE
UTM Zone (WGS84) 13S
Easting 0332213.4
Northing 4073673.5
Latitude 36° 47' 38.51"
Longtitude 106° 52 '50.17"
Elevation: 7,687 feet

MUNDO LAKE
UTM Zone (WGS84) 13S
Easting 0327911.1
Northing 4082926.5
Latitude 36° 52' 35.85"
Longtitude 106° 55' 51.17"
Elevation: 7,296 feet

STONE LAKE
(north entrance)
UTM Zone (WGS84) 13S
Easting 0332121.4
Northing 4066496.4
Latitude 36° 43' 45.65"
Longtitude 106° 52' 48.17"
Elevation: 7,275

> *Lush green meadows are filled with wildflowers, grazing cattle, and herds of elk.*

LOCATED **20** MILES WEST OF **T**RES **P**IEDRAS, Hopewell Lake is located along the 48-mile stretch of NM 64 connecting Tres Piedras and Tierra Amarilla. Sections of this highway are closed in winter. This is among the prettiest and most scenic drives in the nation. Rolling mountains of blue and edelmann spruce, ponderosa pine, douglas and white fir mix with aspen trees. The lush green meadows are filled with wildflowers, grazing cattle, and herds of elk. This area makes a magnificent photographer's paradise. You will see some aspen groves defoliated along NM 64. These trees died as a result of an infestation of western tent caterpillars, with past drought conditions contributing to their demise. Western tent caterpillars are widespread throughout the forests of the southwest, and 35,800 acres fell victim in New Mexico alone. Despite the outbreak, the aspens within Hopewell Lake Campground are surviving nicely, and the area is still incredibly beautiful.

Hopewell Lake has two areas; the lake area and the campground. The lake area is day use only. This road is quite bumpy as it descends the hill to the parking areas at the lakeside. The host's campsite is at the lake entrance. The lake itself is small, only 25 water acres. The State of New Mexico stocks the lake with rainbow trout, and the fishing is generally good. There are more than 20 picnic tables along the lakeshore, with a large shelter reserved for group picnics. Two modern vault toilets with water spigots and trash receptacles are provided at the lakeside and shelter.

Hopewell Lake Campground was originally dispersed camping with no amenities. The camp was closed several years and reopened in 2003. The original campground road has been graveled. With 32 campsites, the one loop is quite large, with four modern vault toilets. Trash receptacles and a water spigot

RATINGS

Beauty: ✿ ✿ ✿ ✿ ✿
Privacy: ✿ ✿ ✿ ✿
Spaciousness: ✿ ✿ ✿ ✿
Quiet : ✿ ✿ ✿
Security: ✿ ✿ ✿
Cleanliness: ✿ ✿ ✿ ✿

are located at each toilet location. The well is deep, providing cold sweet water that should be filtered. Most sites are well spaced, private, and very shady. Sites 16, 17, 18, and 22 are in an open meadow and have no shade. Most sites are large.

Campsites 16 and 17 are reserved for equestrian campers and have no shade. Trail riders and hikers have three different trails to explore. The trailheads are located across from campsite 10, between campsites 15 and 16, and a gated access road between 16 and 17. The ruins of the old mining town of Hopewell can be explored. The remains are located to the west of the lake on the hillside.

All campsites have a new picnic table and fire ring. The ground is dirt, but there are many grassy areas to pitch tents. The campsites most appealing to tent campers are 19 through 32. RVs tend to prefer campsites 1 through 15. The RV-to-tent ratio is about 50/50 at this campground, but with adequate distance between the sites, there is little interference. No generator use restrictions exist at this campground. There is plenty of firewood, mostly aspen, within the camp and in adjacent forest areas.

Hopewell Lake Campground is less than 20 miles as the crow flies to the border of Colorado. The elevation is more than 9,800 feet high. Prepare for warm days in the 80s and cold nights in the 40s. Thunderstorms are common in this area, so be prepared to take shelter. Black bear, mountain lion, and bobcat are common; rein in the kids and pets.

The camp is patrolled by the Forest Service. New Mexico Game Wardens check licenses and provide some security for the campground. Rio Arriba County Sheriff Department officers may make occasional stops at this camp.

KEY INFORMATION

ADDRESS: Tres Piedras Ranger District P.O. Box 38 Tres Piedras, NM 87113 (505) 758-8678 Office on the north side of NM 64, west of Tres Piedras www.fs.fed.us/r3/carson/index.shtml

OPERATED BY: Tres Piedras Ranger District Carson National Forest U.S. Department of Agriculture

OPEN: Mid-May–mid-September, weather permitting

SITES: 32 individual sites; all sites are first come, first served

EACH SITE HAS: Parking space, picnic table, and fire ring

REGISTRATION: Self-service registration, immediately upon selecting campsite

FEE: $10 per night single unit

ELEVATION: 9,850 feet

RESTRICTIONS: *Pets:* On leash, 6-foot maximum; take precautionary measures for predators *Fires:* Wood fires permitted in fire rings; charcoal grills are permitted *Alcohol:* Within campsite only *Quiet Hours:* 10 p.m.–8 a.m. *Stay Limit:* 14 days

MAP

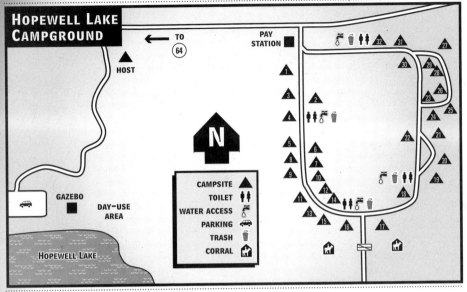

HOPEWELL LAKE CAMPGROUND

TO 64

PAY STATION

HOST

N

GAZEBO
DAY-USE AREA

HOPEWELL LAKE

CAMPSITE	▲
TOILET	
WATER ACCESS	
PARKING	
TRASH	
CORRAL	

GETTING THERE

From Tres Piedras, drive west on NM 64 for 20 miles. The lake is viewable from the roadside, and there is a sign. Drive up the road past the lake entrance road, and the campground entrance is another 50 yards on the right.

GPS COORDINATES

UTM Zone 13S
Easting 0389820
Northing 4062471
Latitude 36° 42' 05.5"
Longtitude 106° 14' 0.5"

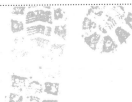

NORTHEAST CAMPGROUNDS:
Carson National Forest

05
COLUMBINE
CAMPGROUND

T IS IRONIC THAT ONE OF New Mexico's most majestic campgrounds sits right across the highway from one of the state's worst environmental disasters. Columbine Campground is located across the highway from the Molycorp Molybdenum Mine. The ugly mining scars will remain upon these mountains for thousands of years, and they may be viewed from this camp.

That being said, this campground is one of the loveliest in New Mexico. The campground sits in a dense growth of ponderosa pine, spruce, fir, aspen, and cottonwood. Tiny Columbine Creek runs through this campground, and if you select campsite numbers 15, 17, 18, 26, or 27, you will be the closest to this delightful meandering stream. Columbine Creek flows into Red River by the camp's entrance bridge. It is an easy walk downhill to fish the river. New Mexico Fish and Game officers check for licenses and possession limits regularly.

Columbine Campground is less rocky and more grassy than the Red River campgrounds profiled in this book. It is not as popular either, which is a benefit for those who value privacy. Columbine is a tent-camper's paradise, but you can expect a few RVs. The campground traffic increases on weekends due to the Columbine trailhead that begins in the camp. Predators are common here, so watch children closely and keep your pets leashed.

The ice truck visits Columbine and delivers ice for the same price as local stores. There is no firewood to gather at Columbine, but a gentleman in a truck sells a box for $5. Firewood is also for sale in the towns of Questa and Red River.

Red River is 5.8 miles east and Questa is 5.2 miles west of Columbine. Red River is much more appealing to visit than Questa, but both towns offer

> *One of the loveliest campgrounds in New Mexico.*

RATINGS

Beauty: ✪ ✪ ✪ ✪ ✪
Privacy: ✪ ✪ ✪
Spaciousness: ✪ ✪ ✪
Quiet: ✪ ✪ ✪
Security: ✪ ✪ ✪ ✪ ✪
Cleanliness: ✪ ✪ ✪ ✪ ✪

ADDRESS: Carson National
Forest
Questa Ranger
District
P.O. Box 110
Questa, NM 87556
(505) 586-0520 or
758-6230; www.fs
.fed.us/r3/carson

OPERATED BY: Questa Ranger
District
Carson National
Forest
U.S. Department
of Agriculture

OPEN: Official season,
May 1–October 15

SITES: 27 individual sites;
all sites are first
come, first served

EACH SITE HAS: Parking space, picnic
table, and fire ring

REGISTRATION: Self-service
registration,
immediately upon
selecting campsite

FEE: $15 per night single
unit

ELEVATION: 8,041 feet

RESTRICTIONS: *Pets:* On leash, 6-foot
maximum; take
precautionary
measures for
predators
Fires: Wood fires
permitted only in
provided fire rings;
charcoal grills are
permitted
Alcohol: Within
campsite only
Quiet Hours: 10 p.m.–
8 a.m.
Stay Limit: 14 days

full-service grocery stores, gas stations, and fishing and camping supplies.

In years past, no campground host has been assigned here. The Forest Service, New Mexico Fish and Game, and Taos County Sheriff's Departments patrol this campground frequently. Plans are underway to assign a host here.

Because of the topography of the campground, road noise impacts Columbine little, and the campground sits back from the highway. Because Columbine is nearly 800 feet lower in altitude, the weather is somewhat warmer than Red River camps. The snowfall here is less and the Forest Service opens up this campground three weeks earlier than the Red River locations.

The Columbine Canyon Trailhead begins on the back side of the campground. The trailhead has its own parking area. The trailhead follows a gentle grade up Columbine Canyon. It is popular with hikers and is rated easy to moderate. Access to the creek, wildflower-filled meadows, and occasional views of the high mountains to the south make this an ideal trail. Nearby, Goat Hill Campground is adjacent to NM 38 on the south side of the highway and isn't nearly as appealing as the other campgrounds nearby. The campground is shady but directly on the highway. The ground is crushed gravel and better suited to trailers and small RVs than to tents. La Bobita Campground across the road is much more appealing to campers than Goat Hill, but is opened rarely.

MAP

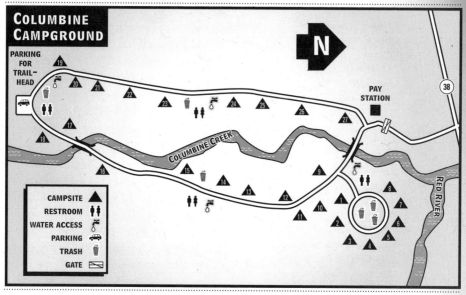

COLUMBINE CAMPGROUND

PARKING FOR TRAIL-HEAD

N

PAY STATION

38

COLUMBINE CREEK

RED RIVER

CAMPSITE	▲
RESTROOM	🚹🚺
WATER ACCESS	🚰
PARKING	🚗
TRASH	🗑
GATE	▱

GETTING THERE

From Questa, Turn East and follow Highway 38 5.8 miles; Turn Right into campground at sign.

GPS COORDINATES

UTM Zone (WGS84) 13S
Easting 0453939
Northing 4059568
Latitude 36° 40' 50.3"
Longtitude 105° 30' 55.1"

06
ELEPHANT ROCK CAMPGROUND

> *Set up on a hillside, this lovely campground is beautifully terraced with large campsites.*

ELEPHANT ROCK CAMPGROUND is across NM 38 from Fawn Lakes, an easy one-half mile walk to Fawn Lakes Campground. Set up on a hillside, this lovely campground is beautifully terraced, with large campsites. Elephant Rock offers the privacy that Junebug or Fawn Lakes campgrounds do not provide. This camp is often overlooked by those who prefer riverside camping and is the last campground nearest to the town of Red River to fill up on the weekends. This campground provides the best seclusion of all of the Red River campgrounds. Most sites are large enough to accommodate two or more tents and spaced a significant distance away from one another.

The forest here is a mix of ponderosa, spruce, fir, and aspen. The hillside is rocky. The large stone-terraced campsites are level and provide good water runoff. When it rains here, it can be a real gully washer.

You will see a few RVs here. The views looking across the highway over the Red River Valley and the mountain range to the south are lovely. Behind this campground, the trees thin significantly to reveal Elephant Rock, at its 10,556-foot elevation. The hillside becomes very steep and due to loose rock can be a hazard to climbers.

The campground has four water spigots, two located on each end of the loop and two in the center of the campground. Water is supplied from the city of Red River pumping station. The water is cold and sweet. There are three vault toilets, located at each end and center of the grounds. These facilities are nearly new and are extremely well maintained. The entire campground is very clean. There may be an occasional bear or coyote in the camp, but bears tend to spend more time along the river, across the highway. You may see occasional mule deer.

While driving down NM State Highway 38,

RATINGS

Beauty: ✿ ✿ ✿ ✿ ✿
Privacy: ✿ ✿ ✿ ✿
Spaciousness: ✿ ✿ ✿ ✿
Quiet: ✿ ✿ ✿ ✿
Security: ✿ ✿ ✿ ✿ ✿
Cleanliness: ✿ ✿ ✿ ✿ ✿

watch closely for pedestrians, bicycles, and vehicles. It is advisable to beware of wildlife crossing the highway. This is a busy highway during camping season, but surprisingly the campground gets very little road noise from the highway. Elephant Rock is safe for children, and there are no water hazards in the camp. The center of the campground gives kids some running room and the loop is fun for bicycling. The Red River has excellent fishing; just walk across the highway.

Regular patrols are made by the Forest Service and Taos County Sheriff's Departments, and the security here is very good. Your cellular phone may not pick up a signal at this camp.

As with all Red River Campgrounds, the ice truck stops by regularly on weekends. The host usually sells wood at $3 per bundle.

KEY INFORMATION

ADDRESS: Carson National Forest Questa Ranger District P.O. Box 110 Questa, NM 87113 505) 586-0520 or 758-6230; www.fs.fed.us/r3/carson

OPERATED BY: Questa Ranger District Carson National Forest U.S. Department of Agriculture

OPEN: Official season, the weekend before Memorial Day–weekend after Labor Day

SITES: 22 individual sites; all sites are first come, first served

EACH SITE HAS: Parking space, picnic table, and fire ring

REGISTRATION: Self-service registration, immediately upon selecting campsite

FEE: $15 per night single unit

ELEVATION: 8,431 feet

RESTRICTIONS: *Pets:* On leash, 6-foot maximum; take precautionary measures for predators
Fires: Wood fires permitted only in provided fire rings; charcoal grills are permitted
Alcohol: Within campsite only
Quiet Hours: 10 p.m.–8 a.m.
Stay Limit: 14 days

MAP

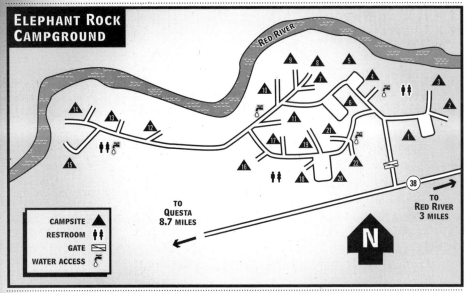

GETTING THERE

From Questa, turn east on NM 38 and drive 8.7 miles. Turn north into the campground.

GPS COORDINATES

UTM Zone (WGS84) 13S
Easting 0459301
Northing 4062340
Latitude 36° 42' 21.1"
Longtitude 105° 27' 20.4"

07
FAWN LAKES CAMPGROUND

FAWN LAKES IS A BEAUTIFUL campground just 3.5 miles from Red River and, like nearby Junebug Campground, fills quickly most weekends. Fawn Lakes will attract RVs, but it is ideal for tent camping. If you select a riverside campsite, you can pitch your tent close to the river for more privacy. The river can be heard throughout the campground, and flows 25 to 50 cubic feet per second during the camping season.

Fawn Lakes campground sits deeply entrenched in the Red River Valley, encapsulated by mountains on both sides. In the summer, daytime temperatures may reach 80°F. Evening temperatures drop quickly, so bring a warm jacket. Nighttime mercury may drop below 40°F, so bring warm sleeping bags.

Located right off NM 38, some traffic noise can be heard at the sites close to the highway. If you camp close to the river, you will never hear it. Fawn Lakes is very shady, with spruce, fir, ponderosa, aspen, cottonwood, and river willow. Fishing is exceptional here, and the river is regularly stocked by the Red River Hatchery located 8 miles southwest of Questa.

The riverside campsites are spacious. Off the end loop, three tent sites are available. You must pack away your food items at night due to bears. There are two toilets, one located at the entrance and one located near the loop. This entire campground is very clean. Fawn Lakes has three water spigots, one at each end of the loop and the other at the center of the loop.

Picnic table and fire grates are provided at all sites. Stage II fire restrictions can go into effect from campground opening until the monsoon season begins in July.

This is black bear country, so abide by the posted bear alerts, and you will be safe. Coyotes are common around this area, too, so rein in your children and pets.

> *Deeply entrenched in the Red River Valley, encapsulated by mountains on both sides*

RATINGS

Beauty: ✰ ✰ ✰ ✰
Privacy: ✰ ✰
Spaciousness: ✰ ✰ ✰
Quiet: ✰ ✰ ✰
Security: ✰ ✰ ✰ ✰ ✰
Cleanliness: ✰ ✰ ✰ ✰ ✰

KEY INFORMATION

ADDRESS: Questa Ranger District Carson National Forest P.O. Box 110 Questa, NM 87113 (505) 586-0520 or 758-6320; www.fs .fed.us/r3/carson

OPERATED BY: Questa Ranger District Carson National Forest U.S. Department of Agriculture

OPEN: Opens 1 week before Memorial Day weekend, closes 1 week after Labor Day weekend

SITES: 22 individual sites; all sites are first come, first served

EACH SITE HAS: Parking space, picnic table, and fire ring

REGISTRATION: Self-service registration, immediately upon selecting campsite

FEE: $10 per night single unit

ELEVATION: 8,515 feet

RESTRICTIONS: *Pets:* On leash, 6-foot maximum; take precautionary measures for predators
Fires: Wood fires permitted only in provided fire rings; charcoal grills are permitted
Alcohol: Within campsite only
Quiet Hours: 10 p.m.– 8 a.m.
Stay Limit: 14 days

Raccoons can be heard every night, so lock the food in your vehicle. There are no bear-proof food lockers provided here.

Broad-tailed hummingbird (*Selasphorus platycercus*) and the Rufous hummingbird (*Selasphorus rufus*) are residents at this campground. Put away your feeder at night, though, because it will attract bears.

A campground host is here; the Forest Service, New Mexico Game and Fish Department, and Taos County Sheriff's Department patrol frequently. Fishing license and possession checks are conducted frequently, so beware.

Kids love Fawn Lakes, and there is much to keep them busy here. The three ponds called Fawn Lakes are an easy walk west of the campground. Ducks in the pond are fun to feed and photograph. The ponds have hiking trails that are a blast on a mountain bike.

This campground is somewhat quieter than Junebug. Anglers may intrude near riverside campsites.

Two ladies sell block and cube ice out of their truck on weekends; you might tip them. A gentleman sells firewood from his truck on weekends, and the campground host sells firewood for $3 a bundle.

Red River is a fun town with numerous restaurants and stores. Several saloons serve food and offer live bands on the weekends. Several outfitter stores cater to campers and anglers. Der Markt Grocery is a full-service store, and prices are reasonable. Cellular service is available in Red River, and cell phones work at Fawn Lakes Campground. Free wireless high-speed Internet service is available at the new conference center just behind the park on Main Street. Internet service is free at the Chamber of Commerce building. Try Texas Red's Steakhouse for a buffalo burger or a steak.

Many activities abound throughout the Red River Valley. Jeeps and ATVs can be rented in town and four-wheel-drive vehicle tours are available. Horseback riding is available here. There are hundreds of acres the Mallette Canyon Access road is a must for ATV and four-wheel drive enthusiasts.

The Circle of Enchantment drive covers 85 miles. The drive encompasses some of the prettiest vistas in the United States. Visit Taos, Taos Pueblo, and Taos

MAP

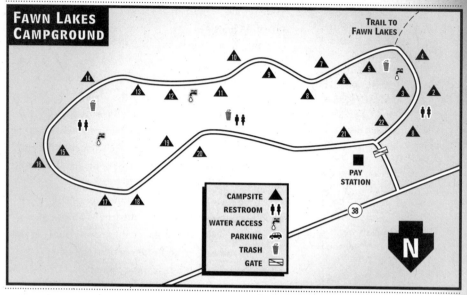

FAWN LAKES CAMPGROUND

TRAIL TO FAWN LAKES

PAY STATION

38

N

CAMPSITE	▲	
RESTROOM	♂♀	
WATER ACCESS		
PARKING	🚗	
TRASH	🗑	
GATE	⬛	

Mountain Casino. The Vietnam Memorial near the town of Angel Fire is a must, and the town and lake of Eagle Nest and the ghost town of Elizabethtown both have worthwhile attractions.

GETTING THERE

From Taos, go north on NM 522 to town of Questa. Turn east on NM 38 9.3 miles and turn into the campground on your right.

GPS COORDINATES

UTM Zone (WGS84) 13S
Easting 0459870
Northing 4062511
Latitude 36° 42' 26.7"
Longtitude 105° 26' 57.5"

> *There is no campground like Junebug!*

THERE IS NO PLACE LIKE RED RIVER, New Mexico, and there is no campground like Junebug. I've been coming here since 1991. This pretty campground is just 2 miles from Red River and fills most weekends. Junebug gets a few RVs, but you'll find great tent camping here. Pick a riverside campsite and pitch the tent close to the river. The Forest Service has planned an extensive renovation of this campground; the water system will be improved, a new vault toilet will be installed, the host site will have an electrical hookup, and the gravel road will be covered with asphalt.

The river can be heard throughout the campground and flows between 25 to 50 cubic feet per second during the camping season. In 2005 and 2006, the river overflowed its banks and flooded half of the riverside campsites.

The Red River Valley is deeply entrenched by mountains on both sides. In the summer it rarely exceeds 80°F. When a cold front comes in, the temperature can drop rapidly, so bring a warm jacket. Night time temperatures may drop below 40°F, so pack warm sleeping bags.

Junebug is very shady, with a mixture of spruce, fir, ponderosa, aspen, cottonwood, and river willow. Fishing is exceptional here, stocked regularly by the hatchery located southwest of Questa. On our maiden trip here, our 8-year-old son caught our limit of trout before his mother and I got the camp set up.

You will notice the riverside campsites are quite spacious. The ground may be rocky in places, so bring a thick ground pad. There are two toilets, one located across from campsite 4, and a brand-new facility located on the end loop. This entire campground is extremely clean. Two water spigots serve Junebug, one at the entry and another across from campsite 2. The

RATINGS

Beauty: ✪ ✪ ✪ ✪
Privacy: ✪
Spaciousness: ✪ ✪ ✪ ✪
Quiet: ✪
Security: ✪ ✪ ✪ ✪ ✪
Cleanliness: ✪ ✪ ✪ ✪ ✪

water is icy cold and sweet and comes from the city pumping station across the highway.

Each campsite comes with a picnic table and fire grate. Springtime is usually fairly dry, and Stage II fire restrictions may go into effect until July when the monsoon season begins. Don't let that discourage you, though; come up and cold camp. The forest has a lovely fragrance that is masked by wood smoke.

This is serious black bear country, and bears are occasionally spotted in town. Abide by the posted bear alerts, and you won't get on their list. Mountain lion and bobcat won't venture this close to the town of Red River. A coyote was spotted across the river from the camp, though, so rein in your pets. Raccoons are quite common at Junebug, trying to get into mischief every night.

Hummingbirds love this campground, so bring your feeder. The most common species here are the broad-tailed hummingbird (*Selasphorus platycercus*) and the Rufous hummingbird (*Selasphorus rufus*). They provide all-day entertainment and are easy to photograph. Put away your feeder at night, however, because it will attract bears and raccoons.

The campground has a host assigned here, and the Forest Service patrols regularly, as well as the New Mexico Game and Fish Department and Taos County Sheriff's Department. Have your fishing license with you because license and possession checks are frequent here.

The Memorial Day Red River Rally attracts more than 10,000 motorcycle riders. The town is built for 2,000. If you are a tent-packing Harley rider, you'll enjoy this campground.

Privacy and quiet on weekends is hard to find, so try to plan weekday camping. Anglers inevitably pass near your riverside campsite, but overall the campers here are courteous and respectful.

Every weekend a truck comes by and sells ice at the same price as in town. I usually tip them. The campground host sells firewood for $3 a bundle. There are no firewood gathering areas nearby.

Red River is a friendly town, with an ice cream shop, restaurants, and shopping. Several stores cater to

KEY INFORMATION

ADDRESS: Questa Ranger District Carson National Forest P.O. Box 110 Questa, NM 87113 (505) 586-0520 or 758-6320; www.fs.fed.us/r3/carson

OPERATED BY: Questa Ranger District Carson National Forest U.S. Department of Agriculture

OPEN: Opens 1 week before Memorial Day weekend, closes 1 week after Labor Day weekend

SITES: 20 individual sites; all sites are first come, first served

EACH SITE HAS: Parking space, picnic table, and fire ring

REGISTRATION: Self-service registration, immediately upon selecting campsite

FEE: $15 per night single unit

ELEVATION: 8,586 feet

RESTRICTIONS: *Pets:* On leash, 6-foot maximum; take precautionary measures for predators
Fires: Wood fires permitted only in provided fire rings; charcoal grills permitted
Alcohol: Within campsite only
Quiet Hours: 10 p.m.–8 a.m.
Stay Limit: 14 days

MAP

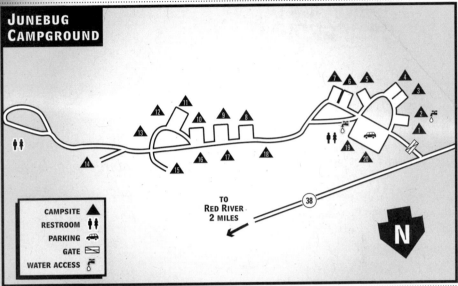

JUNEBUG CAMPGROUND

CAMPSITE ▲
RESTROOM 👫
PARKING 🚗
GATE ✉
WATER ACCESS 🚰

TO
RED RIVER
2 MILES

38

N

GETTING THERE

From Taos, go north on NM 522 to town of Questa. Turn east on NM 38 for 11 miles and turn into the campground on your right.

campers and anglers. Der Markt Grocery is a full-service grocery, and prices are reasonable.

You can ride the chairlift to the top of the ski area. From there, hiking trails lead to the summit of New Mexico's highest mountain, Wheeler Peak. The Circle of Enchantment drive is 85 miles long. The drive features the cultural town of Taos, the Taos Pueblo, Taos Casino, the Vietnam Memorial in the town of Angel Fire, the town and lake of Eagle Nest, and the ghost town of Elizabethtown.

GPS COORDINATES

UTM Zone (WGS84) 13S
Easting 461106
Northing 4062610
Latitude 36° 42' 30.8"
Longtitude 105° 26' 13.3"

WHEN **LOUIS L'AMOUR** wrote his novel *The Sacketts*, he admitted his inability to describe the beauty of the Mora Valley. Words cannot do it justice. You have to experience it for yourself. Surrounded by ponderosa pine–covered mountains, this lush valley is filled with green pasture lands of cattle and horses grazing in the cool mountain breezes. This valley is old; dozens of crumbling adobe homes give testimony to the pioneers who tamed this majestic land. Several alpaca ranches in the area raise herds of these docile animals, and stores in the area sell alpaca wool products. These are the things that you experience driving north from the town of Mora to Coyote Creek State Park.

Coyote Creek State Park is 17 miles north of the town of Mora. Coyote Creek is a premier tent-camper's park with 47 campsites. Reserved RV campsites are clustered together just past the comfort station, with electric and water hookups provided, separating the sought-after RV sites from the rest of the park.

A large meadow runs the length of the park, deep with native grasses and abounding in wildflowers. A modern playground in the meadow stays busy all day. Two campsites sit on top of the hill up a short dirt road. Both sites are equipped with an Adirondack shelter, picnic table, and fire rings.

Seven more campsites adjacent to the playground are large, well spaced, and private. Four of these seven sites are equipped with Adirondack shelters; the other three are under trees and shady. These sites can be used by either tents or RVs. These sites are reasonably level and the ground is grassy, ideal for tents.

The road continues through the meadow and across a bridge. Several campsites are along the roadway, with shelters that will catch dust. The RV dump

> *The park explodes in colors . . . oak trees, river willows, and ponderosa pine greenery.*

RATINGS

Beauty: ✿ ✿ ✿ ✿ ✿
Privacy: ✿ ✿ ✿ ✿
Spaciousness: ✿ ✿ ✿ ✿
Quiet: ✿ ✿ ✿ ✿ ✿
Security: ✿ ✿ ✿ ✿ ✿
Cleanliness: ✿ ✿ ✿ ✿ ✿

ADDRESS: Coyote Creek State Park
P.O. Box 477
Guadalupita, NM 87722
www.emnrd.state.nm.us/PRD/CoyoteCreek.htm

OPERATED BY: New Mexico State Parks

OPEN: Year-round. In winter, water may not be available and park may be inaccessible; call ahead for details.

SITES: 47 individual sites; 7 sites are reserveable; the remaining sites are first come, first served

EACH SITE HAS: Parking space, picnic table, and fire ring; 9 sites are equipped with Adirondack shelters

REGISTRATION: Self-service registration, immediately upon selecting campsite

FEE: $10 per night single unit

ELEVATION: 7,772 feet

RESTRICTIONS: *Pets:* On leash, 6-foot maximum; take precautionary measures for predators
Fires: Wood fires permitted only in fire rings; charcoal grills are permitted
Alcohol: Within campsite only; no glass permitted
Quiet Hours: 10 p.m.–8 a.m.
Stay Limit: 14 days

station is located here. More tent sites are up the hill; these sites sit among gambel oak, pinon, cedar, and ponderosa pines. The sites are dirt and have no grass, but provide great tent camping with a great view. These sites are closer together, but private due to the undergrowth of young trees and oak bushes.

All sites are equipped with a fire ring and picnic table. Five modern vault toilets are distributed throughout the park and are kept very clean. The visitor center at the entrance is equipped with a spotless comfort station with sinks, flush toilets, and a shower. The small office is open occasionally with trail maps and state park information brochures.

One hiking trail circles the park, featuring foot bridges, benches, an old moonshiner's shack, and a cold-water spring piped into a hewn-log livestock watering trough. The trail is 1.5 miles in length, and is more like a leisurely walk than a hike. Beware of nettles and poison ivy in the deep grass. Due to recent rains, the trail is overgrown with knee-high vegetation. The trail is alive with wildflowers from spring to fall, providing a photographer with dozens of species. The park explodes in colors in the fall with oak trees and river willows providing the show, set among the ponderosa pine greenery.

For anglers, Coyote Creek is the most densely stocked water in New Mexico. Twelve- to 15-inch rainbow trout are common. Within the park boundaries are two beaver ponds that provide excellent fishing spots along the stream. The fish are brought in several times a year from the Mora Fish Hatchery.

At night, the surrounding mountains are dimly silhouetted by the town lights of Mora to the south and Angel Fire to the north; yet the sky is pitch black and makes Coyote Creek a perfect place for stargazing.

Many birds are endemic to the park, and you can spot various raptors riding the air currents to the east over the mountain ridges. Black bear, mountain lion, bobcat, elk, mule deer, beaver, raccoon, skunk, and badger make their homes in the surrounding mountains; and coyote can be heard singing every night.

MAP

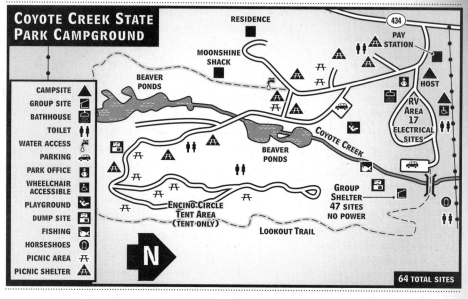

COYOTE CREEK STATE PARK CAMPGROUND

RESIDENCE

434

PAY STATION

MOONSHINE SHACK

BEAVER PONDS

HOST

RV AREA 17 ELECTRICAL SITES

COYOTE CREEK

BEAVER PONDS

GROUP SHELTER 47 SITES NO POWER

ENCINO CIRCLE TENT AREA (TENT ONLY)

LOOKOUT TRAIL

N

CAMPSITE	
GROUP SITE	
BATHHOUSE	
TOILET	
WATER ACCESS	
PARKING	
PARK OFFICE	
WHEELCHAIR ACCESSIBLE	
PLAYGROUND	
DUMP SITE	
FISHING	
HORSESHOES	
PICNIC AREA	
PICNIC SHELTER	

64 TOTAL SITES

GETTING THERE

From Mora, New Mexico, turn right at the Coyote Creek State Park sign onto NM 434 for 17 miles. The park turnoff is on the right.

GPS COORDINATES

UTM Zone (WGS84) 13S
Easting 0478891
Northing 4003717
Latitude 36° 10' 40.8"
Longtitude 105° 14' 05.1"

10
MORPHY LAKE
STATE PARK
CAMPGROUND

> *One of the best primitive tent-camping parks in New Mexico*

BEAUTIFUL **MORPHY LAKE STATE PARK** is one of the best primitive tent-camping parks in New Mexico. Morphy Lake was accessible only by four-wheel-drive for many years, but the road was paved in the spring of 2007. The entry road remains extremely steep in parts, with twists and turns—not for the faint of heart. Once word gets out that the road is paved, this campground will stay full.

Morphy Lake is open year-round for ice fishing, and the campground is open from April 1 to November 1. Snow begins to fall as early as October, and winter storms are possible through late April. No snow removal is performed on this road. Off-season campers and anglers are encouraged to call ahead for road and weather conditions.

At the park entrance, a sign indicates trailers are limited to 18 feet due to tight turn-arounds. Pop-up campers are common here. Little Morphy Lake is a pretty blue mountain lake with 15 water acres, and the park is just 30 land acres. Within its boundaries are 20 campsites. The campsites circle the northern half of the lake. One hiking trail encircles the lake.

Each campsite is equipped with a fire ring and a picnic table. Shade is excellent here, provided by a healthy ponderosa pine forest. The campsites are not large, but each site can accommodate any size tent, and sites are fairly level and reasonably spaced apart. All campsites have a spectacular view of the lake. The campsites are dirt; there is no grass. All sites are along the road, and dust can be stirred up by either cars or wind.

To the west, views of 13,103-foot Trampas and 12,175-foot Truchas peaks are spectacular, and 12,500-foot Pecos Baldy can be seen as well. Snow is visible above timberline much of the year. Shoreline photos

RATINGS

Beauty: ☆ ☆ ☆ ☆ ☆
Privacy: ☆ ☆ ☆
Spaciousness: ☆ ☆ ☆
Quiet: ☆ ☆ ☆ ☆
Security: ☆ ☆ ☆ ☆ ☆
Cleanliness: ☆ ☆ ☆ ☆ ☆

are best taken in the morning, with the peaks in the background.

There are five clean vault toilets equally spaced throughout the campground. There is no potable water here; you must bring in your own. There is no refuse collection either, so you must pack out your trash. There is no firewood because the forest has been picked clean. Water and firewood are for sale in Mora, 11.5 miles away. Mora has several gas stations, a few cafes, a liquor store, and a full-service grocery with limited camping and picnic supplies.

This lake is great for canoes, kayaks, and inflatable boats, powered by paddle or electric trolling motors only. There is a concrete boat-launch ramp. The lake is regularly stocked with trout from the Mora Fish Hatchery. A fishing tournament is held each August when the lake is filled with 600 20- to 22-inch rainbow trout.

Due to the park's remote location, black bears are common. Stowing all food and trash in your vehicle at night is not an option; bear-proof storage boxes are not provided. Raccoons are common, too, and chipmunks scurry all over the camp. Bring your hummingbird feeder because the little creatures are abundant. Elk, mule deer, skunk, badger, mountain lion, bobcat, and coyote reside in the forests nearby. A free coyote concert begins every morning between 3 a.m. and 5 a.m. Afternoon thunderstorms are common and potentially violent, with lightning.

KEY INFORMATION

ADDRESS: Morphy Lake State Park
P.O. Box 477
Guadalupita, NM 87722
www.emnrd.state
.nm.us/PRD/
MorphyLake.htm

OPERATED BY: New Mexico State Parks

OPEN: Official season, April 1–November 1

SITES: 21 individual sites; all sites are first come, first serve

EACH SITE HAS: Parking space, picnic table, and fire ring

REGISTRATION: Self-service registration, immediately upon selecting campsite

FEE: $10 per night single unit

ELEVATION: 8,057 feet

RESTRICTIONS: *Pets:* On leash, 6-foot maximum; take precautionary measures for predators
Fires: Wood fires permitted only in provided fire rings; charcoal grills are permitted
Alcohol: Within campsite only
Quiet Hours: 10 p.m.–8 a.m.
Stay Limit: 14 days
Other: Glass containers prohibited; pack it in/pack it out refuse policy

MAP

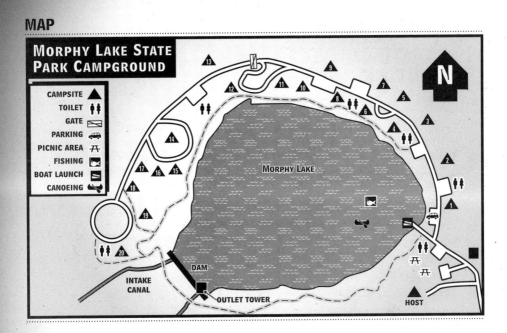

MORPHY LAKE STATE PARK CAMPGROUND

CAMPSITE ▲
TOILET 👫
GATE
PARKING 🚐
PICNIC AREA 🪑
FISHING 🎣
BOAT LAUNCH
CANOEING 🛶

MORPHY LAKE

DAM

INTAKE CANAL

OUTLET TOWER

HOST

GETTING THERE

From Mora, turn south at the Catholic Church onto NM 94 for 7 miles to the town of Ledoux. In Ledoux, turn right at the Morphy Lake sign onto Mora County Road 635, and drive 4 miles west. The road forks; take the right fork at the sign to the campground.

GPS COORDINATES

UTM Zone 13S
Easting 0464316
Northing 3977435
Latitude 35° 56' 26.2"
Longtitude 105° 23' 44.2"

11
SUGARITE CANYON STATE PARK CAMPGROUNDS

SUGARITE CANYON STATE PARK is rated as one of the most magnificent state parks in New Mexico. The park's property borders the state of Colorado. Within its boundaries lie two beautiful lakes, Lake Alice and Lake Maloya. Lake Maloya's northern edge reaches into Colorado. The park elevations range from 6,900 feet at the park entrance to 8,320 feet atop Little Horse Mesa.

Lake Alice is a small lake of three water acres, while Lake Maloya stretches out over 130 acres. Because Lake Maloya is the water supply for the city of Raton, there is no swimming; but sailboats, fishing boats with electric trolling motors, canoes, kayaks, and rafts are allowed. These lakes are well-stocked with rainbow trout.

The park is home to an old coal camp, accessible from a trailhead behind the visitor center. This hike is approximately 1.5 miles and considered moderate to strenuous. Nine other hiking trails are in the park; information and maps are available at the visitor center. Across from the visitor center is the comfort station, with flush toilets and warm water showers. The facilities are kept extremely clean.

Two campgrounds are within Sugarite Canyon State Park. Lake Alice Campground (right across the road from the lake) is ideal for RVs, with water and electrical hookups. This camp is alongside the park road, so road noise is a factor here. All sites are shady but the 16 sites are tightly compacted. Sites 13 through 16 are designated as tent sites and can be reserved.

The Soda Pocket Campground is a totally different environment. The camp turnoff is 1 mile north of Lake Alice. The turnoff is to the left, a well-maintained gravel road curves and switchbacks uphill, gaining 497 feet in elevation. Outside the main campground is a day-use area and a small equestrian camp.

> *Rated as one of the most magnificent state parks in New Mexico*

RATINGS

Beauty: ☆ ☆ ☆ ☆
Privacy: ☆ ☆ ☆ ☆ ☆
Spaciousness: ☆ ☆ ☆ ☆ ☆
Quiet: ☆ ☆ ☆ ☆ ☆
Security: ☆ ☆ ☆ ☆ ☆
Cleanliness: ☆ ☆ ☆ ☆

ADDRESS: Sugarite Canyon State Park HCR 63, Box 386 Raton, NM 87740 (505) 445-5607; www .emnrd.state.nm.us/ PRD/Sugarite.htm

OPERATED BY: New Mexico State Parks

OPEN: Year-round

SITES: Lake Alice: 16 individual sites, 10 reservable sites; remaining 6 sites are first come, first served. Soda Pocket: 25 individual sites; all are first come, first served

EACH SITE HAS: Parking space, picnic table, and fire ring. Some sites have pedestal grills, shade shelters, and bear boxes

REGISTRATION: Self-service registration, immediately upon selecting campsite

FEE: $10 per night single unit

ELEVATION: Lake Alice: 7,142 feet; Soda Pocket entrance road: 7,891 feet

RESTRICTIONS: *Pets:* On leash, strictly enforced; take precautionary measures for predators *Fires:* Wood fires permitted only in provided fire rings; charcoal grills are permitted *Alcohol:* Within camp site only *Quiet Hours:* 10 p.m.– 8 a.m. *Stay Limit:* 14 days *Other:* Glass containers are prohibited

Arriving at Soda Pocket you will find an ideal tent-camper's campground. This campground is on a first-come first-serve basis. Across from the pay station is a large group camp. The main camp begins along a 300-yard-long gravel road, ending in a in a large loop. Many sites are shady under a thickly forested canopy of gambel oak, interspersed with ponderosa pine, juniper, and cedar trees.

Soda Pocket is a perfect campground for tents, with thick native grasses. The majority of the campsites are large and private, with most sites separated with scrub oak and other bushes. There are 25 campsites here, and all sites are level. The campsites that are not under the tree canopy are equipped with steel shelters over the picnic tables. About half of the sites are equipped with bear boxes. Several campsites have pedestal grills and all have one fire ring and picnic table.

RVs are allowed to camp here, but generator use is restricted, and the camp is very quiet. This is a family-friendly campground. The two vault toilets in the camp are clean, but of older design and smell horrible. Due to water quality issues, the water system at Soda Pocket was turned off, but clean water is available at Lake Alice Campground, though filtering is recommended. There is no firewood to be gathered here, so it's best to bring your own.

The campground hosts keep the camp secure, locking the gate at dusk every evening and providing everyone with the gate combination numbers to access the camp. Frequent patrols by park rangers assure your security here.

Bears are abundant. In spring of 2007, a child's hand was bitten by a foraging bear. The bear was destroyed. There are five individual bears known to frequent this camp. If your site has a bear box, use it. If not, pack all food items in your vehicle every night, and keep a clean camp.

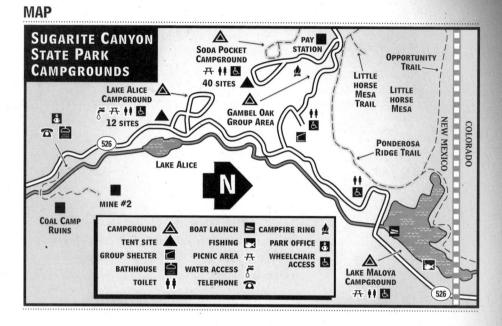

GETTING THERE

From Raton, drive west on NM 72 for 3 miles, turn north on NM 526 and go 2 miles to park entrance. Lake Alice Campground entrance is 0.75 miles north of the park visitor center, and the Soda Pocket Campground road entrance is 1 mile farther north.

GPS COORDINATES

LAKE ALICE CAMPGROUND

UTM Zone (WGS84) 13S

Easting 0554627

Northing 4090472

Latitude 36° 57' 31.5"

Longtitude 104° 23' 11.0"

SODA POCKET CAMPGROUND

UTM Zone (WGS84) 13S

Easting 0554927

Easting 0553850

Northing 4092266

Latitude 36° 58' 29.9"

Longtitude 104° 23' 41.9"

> *Peace, harmony, and two equestrian campgrounds*

VALLE **V**IDAL (in Spanish, meaning Valley of Life) is a lush mountain basin located in the heart of the Sangre de Cristo Mountains of northern New Mexico. Carson National Forest manages this Rocky Mountain paradise. Abundant populations of wildlife, including elk, buffalo, mule deer, black bear, mountain lion, bald eagles, and native Rio Grande cutthroat trout inhabit this protected area. Vast alpine meadows of the Valle Vidal provide critical habitat for the largest herd of elk in New Mexico, numbering more than 2,000 animals.

CIMARRON CAMPGROUND

Beautiful Cimarron Campground is the more pristine of the two campgrounds in Valle Vidal. Surrounded in towering ponderosa pines, aspen, blue spruce, and douglas fir. This lovely place is an equestrian camper's dream come true. There will be some RVs here, but the camp is quiet and majestic. A campground host is assigned here, and frequent ranger and wardens with New Mexico Fish and Game patrol this area frequently.

The campground is divided into two separate loops, with two vault toilets and two water spigots per loop. There are varmint-proof trash receptacles within and outside of the camp. The camp is set up with private roomy sites and some grass. Sites numbered 2, 3, 5 through 11, 13, 20, and 26 through 35 are designated as non-equestrian sites. Those who camp with dogs must keep pets away from the horses. Sites 3 and 17 are designated as wheelchair accessible. Each campsite is equipped with a picnic table and fire ring. Plenty of firewood is available to gather along the roads outside of the camp.

Trails can be used by horses, mountain bikes, or hikers, and there are literally dozens of trails to choose

RATINGS

CIMMARON
Beauty: ✿ ✿ ✿ ✿ ✿
Privacy: ✿ ✿ ✿ ✿
Spaciousness: ✿ ✿ ✿ ✿ ✿
Quiet: ✿ ✿ ✿ ✿
Security: ✿ ✿ ✿ ✿
Cleanliness: ✿ ✿ ✿ ✿

MCCRYSTAL
Beauty: ✿ ✿ ✿ ✿
Privacy: ✿ ✿ ✿ ✿
Spaciousness: ✿ ✿ ✿ ✿
Quiet: ✿ ✿ ✿ ✿
Security: ✿ ✿ ✿
Cleanliness: ✿ ✿ ✿

from, rated from easy to difficult. Nearby, Shuree Ponds are stocked with rainbow trout, and the adjoining Shuree and Ponil Creeks can be fished for Rio Grande cutthroat trout.

This camp is set at more than 9,600 feet elevation, and the temperatures dip into the low 40°F range most nights. Days are mild, never exceeding the mid 80s. Frequent thunderstorms occur here, and lightning is common. Due to its remoteness, black bears frequent this camp; mountain lion and bobcat can be present. Coyote can be heard nearly every night.

KEY INFORMATION

ADDRESS:	Questa Ranger District P.O. Box 10 Questa, NM 87556 (505) 586-0520 Cimmaron: www.fs.fed.us/r3/carson/recreation/camping/cimarron_campground.shtml McCrystal: www.fs.fed.us/r3/carson/recreation/camping/mcCrystal_campground.shtml
OPERATED BY:	Questa Ranger District Carson National Forest U.S. Department of Agriculture
OPEN:	Official season, May 1–November 30, weather permitting. May be opened longer to accommodate hunters.
SITES:	Cimmaron: 36 individual sites; all sites are first come, first served McCrystal: 42 individual sites; all sites are first come, first served
EACH SITE HAS:	Parking space, picnic table, and fire ring; equestrian sites are equipped with corrals and grain bins
REGISTRATION:	Self-service registration, immediately upon selecting campsite
FEE:	Cimmaron: $8 per night single unit. McCrystal: $5 per night single unit
ELEVATION:	Cimmaron: 9,679 feet. McCrystal: 8,144 feet
RESTRICTIONS:	*Pets:* On leash, 6-foot-long maximum; take precautionary measures for predators; keep pets away from horses *Fires:* Wood fires permitted only in provided fire rings; charcoal grills are permitted *Alcohol:* Within campsite only *Quiet Hours:* 10 p.m.–8 a.m. *Stay Limit:* 14 days

MAP

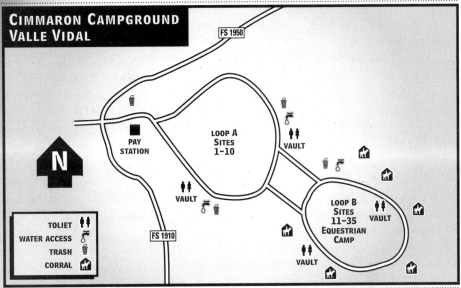

CIMMARON CAMPGROUND
VALLE VIDAL

FS 1950

N

LOOP A
SITES
1-10

PAY
STATION

VAULT

VAULT

LOOP B
SITES
11-35
EQUESTRIAN
CAMP

VAULT

VAULT

FS 1910

TOLIET
WATER ACCESS
TRASH
CORRAL

GETTING THERE

July 1 through end of November: From Costilla, travel east on NM 196 past Amalia, to the intersection of Forest Service 1950. Travel 10 miles on FS 1950 (a gravel road) east to the junction with FS 1910. Cimarron Campground is 1 mile up hill to the right. (This gate is closed during elk calving season, from April 1 through June 30.)

April 1 through July 1: From NM 64, 9 miles east of Cimarron New Mexico, turn north on FS 1950 for 35 miles to FS 1910. (This gate is closed from January 1 through March 1 to prevent stress on wintering elk herds.)

These graveled roads are not maintained during the rainy season and may be passable only with a four-wheel-drive vehicle.

GPS COORDINATES

UTM Zone 13S
Easting 0481637
Northing 4069384
Latitude 36° 46' 12.2"
Longtitude 105° 12' 20.8"

MCCRYSTAL CAMPGROUND

McCrystal Campground is a lovely place for the person who wants to enjoy peace and harmony and enjoys horses and equestrian campers. Set in a tall forest of ponderosa pines and abundant in wildflowers, it's located off FS 1950.

This camp is very large, and all sites are level. Most sites are grassy, shady, and well spaced with plenty of room. Equestrian sites are larger with corrals and grain bins, and marked. This campground boasts more than 60 campsites and is used frequently by the Boy Scouts from nearby Philmont Scout Ranch. It is best to call ahead to Questa Ranger Station before planning a trip, because more than 2,000 scouts use this camp throughout the summer.

There is no potable water here, so you must bring in your own. Several stock tanks supply horses with water, but it is not potable for human use. There is plenty of firewood to gather outside of the campground along the roadway. Security is good, and although there is no host here, the Forest Service patrols this area as well as leaders from the Philmont Scout Ranch.

Each campsite is equipped with a picnic table and fire ring. Four portable toilets service the campground. There is little road noise because, due to the remoteness of this campground, there is very little traffic. All campsites are set back far enough away from the road that dust clouds are not a factor. The campsites are equally spaced apart in three large loops. Due to the level sites, almost all sites are wheelchair accessible; however, the toilet facilities are not.

MAP

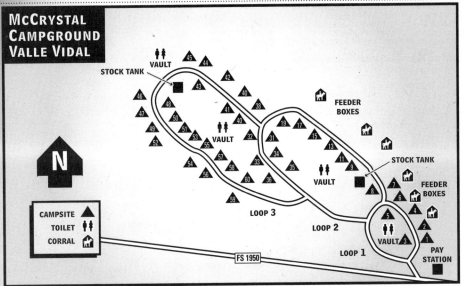

McCrystal Campground Valle Vidal

GETTING THERE

July 1 through end of November: From Costilla, travel east on NM 196 past Amalia, to the intersection of FS 1950. Travel on FS 1950 to the campground approximately 30 miles. (This gate is closed during elk calving season, from April 1 through June 30.)

April 1 through July: 1 From NM 64, travel 9 miles east of Cimarron, New Mexico, turn north on FS 1950 for 35 miles to the campground entrance on the right. (This gate is closed from January 1 through March 1 to prevent stress on wintering elk herds.)

Special Note: These graveled roads are not maintained during the rainy season and may be passable only with a four-wheel-drive vehicle.

GPS COORDINATES

UTM Zone 13S
Easting 0489675
Northing 4070117
Latitude 36° 46' 36.4"
Longtitude 105° 06' 56.5"

NORTH CENTRAL CAMPGROUNDS
SANTA FE NATIONAL FOREST:
Jemez and Cuba Area

13
SAN ANTONIO
CAMPGROUND

> *Families love this campground and there are open areas for children to play.*

A **DELIGHTFUL CAMPGROUND** awaits you just 2 miles north of the small Jemez Mountain community of La Cueva. San Antonio is a tent-camper's delight. Named for San Antonio Creek that flows through this camp, anglers have landed some impressive rainbow trout from this humble little stream.

San Antonio has experienced its share of problems in the past few years, but is still a paradise in its own right. The campground underwent extensive renovation to its water system, only to discover that the water is non potable, containing a high concentration of red volcanic ash. Despite the problems, campers fill this mountain oasis to its brim every weekend between Memorial Day and Labor Day. Potable water is available at Jemez Falls Campground, just a pleasant 5.5-mile drive east on NM 4.

A campground host is assigned to San Antonio; U.S. Forest Service law enforcement officers and the Sandovol County Sheriff's Department patrol this campground frequently, so you will be safe here.

San Antonio has two separate tent areas, totaling 36 campsites. These tent areas are located on each end of the grounds. Several campsites on the north end are handicap accessible; the toilet is equipped with a wheelchair ramp, and there is a wheelchair-accessible fishing spot by the stream.
Four pit toilets are located within an easy walk of all campsites.

The other 11 campsites are individual sites, each with a parking space. The campground is first come, first served, and tent campers are allowed to use individual sites, but you may end up camping next to an RV. Because this is a small campground, privacy is nearly non-existent. Because the campground is right along NM 126, traffic noise can be an irritant.

Despite these drawbacks, the campground is quite

RATINGS

Beauty: ✿ ✿ ✿ ✿
Privacy: ✿
Spaciousness: ✿ ✿
Quiet: ✿
Security: ✿ ✿ ✿ ✿ ✿
Cleanliness: ✿ ✿ ✿

shady with large mature ponderosa pines. Families love this campground, and there are open areas for children to play. The stream is pleasant to fish or soak your feet in. Crossing the stream, several hiking trails wind up the side of the mountain.

This is one of few areas in which mosquitoes are a problem in the Jemez Mountains, so bring insect repellent. On weekends, this campground gets really crowded with traffic. Watch your children and pets carefully.

Another irritant are the nightly raids by raccoons. These masked bandits are not shy at all and are adept at stealing food. Keep all food items in your vehicle. Bears are spotted at this campground every year. I have seen bear tracks by the stream numerous times, so take the necessary precautions, and read and obey the alerts posted at the camp.

The community of La Cueva has a nice little store called Amanda's, stocked with what you might forget to pack from home. The owner, Ray, keeps the prices reasonable. Amanda's carries a good selection of fishing tackle and sells New Mexico fishing licenses. Next door, The Ridgeback Cafe serves great food if you tire of camp cooking. There is no cellular phone service here. The Lewis Realty office next to the cafe has two pay phones.

Hot springs are popular in the Jemez Wilderness. McCauley Warm Springs is a 1.5-mile hike from nearby Battleship Rock picnic grounds. San Antonio Hot Springs is by far the best. From the campground, drive north 3 miles on NM 126, turn off to the right onto Forest Service 376 for 6 bumpy miles. The road ends at the parking lot. Nude bathing is prohibited, and it is a family environment. You will see the large parking area just south of the Rincon Fishing area, a few miles south off NM 4.

KEY INFORMATION

ADDRESS: Jemez Ranger District P.O. Box150 Jemez Springs, NM 87025 (505) 829-3535 www.fs.fed.us/r3/sfe

OPERATED BY: Santa Fe National Forest U.S. Department of Agriculture

OPEN: Official season, Memorial Day–Labor Day

SITES: 47; all sites are first come, first served

EACH SITE HAS: Parking space, picnic table, and fire ring

REGISTRATION: Self-service registration, immediately upon selecting campsite

FEE: $10 per night single unit; $12 per night electrical units (2)

ELEVATION: 8,171 feet

RESTRICTIONS: *Pets:* On leash, 6-foot maximum *Fires:* Wood fires permitted only in provided fire rings; charcoal grills are permitted *Alcohol:* Within campsite only *Quiet Hours:* 10 p.m.– 8 a.m. *Stay Limit:* 14 days

MAP

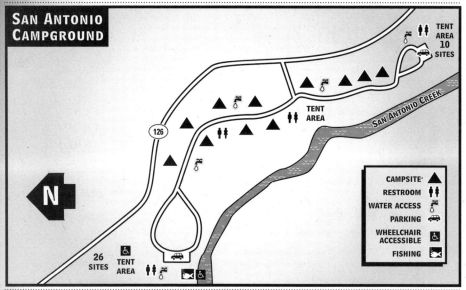

GETTING THERE

From the ranger station in Jemez Springs, drive north on US 4.. Turn left (north) at the La Cueva Junction onto NM 126 and go 2 miles and turn left (east) into the campground.

GPS COORDINATES

UTM Zone (WGS84) 13S
Easting 0351397
Northing 3972571
Latitude N 35° 53' 10.1"
Longtitude W 106° 38' 47.0"

14
REDONDO CAMPGROUND

REDONDO **CAMPGROUND** boasts all the beauty of the Jemez Wilderness you can experience. Encapsulated within a mature forest of tall ponderosa pine, scattered aspen, and other mixed conifers, this campground greets you with the glorious fragrance of the pines. The meadows within Redondo's boundaries fill with wildflowers every spring.

Redondo Campground is close to my heart because it is the first place that I camped after moving to New Mexico in August of 1988. It is the first place my wife, Susan, stepson, Chris, and I camped after our wedding in 1990. Every year I make my pilgrimage back to this lovely environment.

Redondo Campground is named for the 11,254-foot Redondo Peak, visible to the east. Redondo boasts the highest elevation among the Jemez campgrounds at 8,180 feet above sea level, so prepare for summer nights in the 40°F to 50°F range.

Afternoon showers occur frequently during the New Mexico monsoon season beginning in July and continuing through September. Violent lightning storms are common, so be prepared for evasive action. Summer days rarely exceed the mid-80s. Frequent breezes bend the huge ponderosas and perform a beautiful forest symphony.

Redondo Campground is wonderful for children and families. The campground road is exactly 1 mile in length, perfect for a bicycle ride, skateboarding, or a leisurely stroll. Kids love it, and there is plenty of space for them to play.

The Redondo well went dry in 2003, but water is available at Jemez Falls Campground, just 3.5 miles east on NM 4. There is a trace of chlorine in the water, so filtering is wise.

Recent forest thinning for fire protection at this campground has not detracted any beauty from

> *This beautiful campground greets you with the glorious fragrance of pine.*

RATINGS

Beauty: ✿ ✿ ✿ ✿ ✿
Privacy: ✿ ✿ ✿
Spaciousness: ✿ ✿ ✿ ✿
Quiet: ✿ ✿
Security: ✿ ✿ ✿ ✿ ✿
Cleanliness: ✿ ✿ ✿

ADDRESS: Jemez Ranger
District
P.O. Box 150
Jemez Springs, NM
87025
(505) 829-3535
www.fs.fed.us/r3/sfe

OPERATED BY: Santa Fe National
Forest
U.S. Department
of Agriculture

OPEN: Opens early May,
closes mid-
September; official
season, Memorial
Day–Labor Day

SITES: 59; some are
reserveable,
www.reserveusa
.com or call (877)
444-6777; most sites
are first come, first
served

EACH SITE HAS: Parking space, picnic table, and fire
ring

REGISTRATION: Self-service
registration,
immediately upon
selecting campsite

FEE: $10 per night single
unit; $20 per night
double unit

ELEVATION: 8,180 feet

RESTRICTIONS: *Pets:* On leash, 6-foot
maximum, take
precautionay
Fires: Wood fires
permitted only in
provided fire rings;
charcoal grills are
permitted
Alcohol: Within
campsite only
Quiet Hours: 10 p.m.–
8 a.m.

the area, and you will find a significant amount of firewood available.

A campground host is available from Memorial Day through Labor Day. Santa Fe National Forest law enforcement officers and the Sandoval County Sheriff Department patrol frequently. They're strict on policy, but are friendly and helpful. You will be secure at Redondo Campground.

Privacy and spaciousness at this campground will vary. Most of the campsites on the inside of the loops are too closely spaced, whereas the sites on the outside will provide more solitude. RV campers frequent this campground, but there are many places to pitch your tent away from other campers and enjoy your privacy. If you arrive early you will find several campsites that may qualify as "honeymoon suites." All spaces are equipped with a fire ring and picnic table, and most are shaded.

Five pit toilets are distributed conveniently throughout the campground. A fair warning: these facilities are of an old design and are quite putrid as the weather warms.

Flies, bees, and wasps are common in this campground, but there are few mosquitoes or other bloodthirsty pests. You will frequently see many varieties of butterflies. Various species of wood-boring beetles may come for a visit.

If you love hummingbirds, bring your feeder. The New Mexico mountains are home to broadtail hummingbirds. You will also spot rufous hummingbirds, which are territorial and may chase the broadtails off. American crows are residents in the forest here. Blue jays are resident in the campground, as are Stellar's jays.

Deer and elk herds are common in this area, but migrate to remote areas in the Santa Fe National Forest by the time camping season arrives. Be careful driving down NM 4, because wildlife cross this road frequently.

Mule deer, elk, coyote, black bear, mountain lion, and bobcat all make their homes in the surrounding mountain areas. In spring, deer and elk droppings are commonly found within the campground, but they migrate to higher elevations as summer approaches. There have been no reported sightings of predatory

MAP

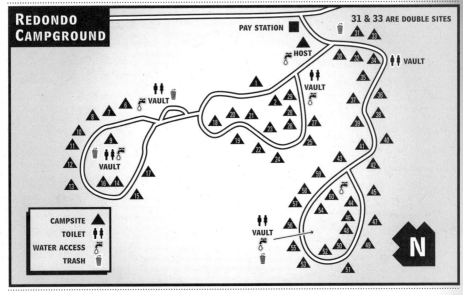

REDONDO CAMPGROUND

PAY STATION

31 & 33 ARE DOUBLE SITES

HOST

VAULT

VAULT

VAULT

VAULT

VAULT

CAMPSITE	▲
TOILET	♦♦
WATER ACCESS	⌐
TRASH	🗑

N

animals within the campgrounds, but be wary because this is black bear country.

There are two hiking and mountain biking trails inside this campground. The Redondo Loop, located within the campground boundaries, is a 2.5-mile round-trip hike. The second trail, the Redondo Campground trail is a 2-mile hike. Both are considered easy to moderate hikes.

Outside of the campground are many forest roads where motorcycles and all-terrain vehicles are permitted. Drive your off-road vehicle carefully; hikers and mountain bikes travel in areas where powered off-road vehicles are permitted. Stop by the Jemez Ranger Station to obtain detailed information regarding motorized vehicles before proceeding and be aware that rules may change frequently.

Redondo Campground has an amphitheater, and it gets a significant amount of use. College students interning with the Forest Service come to give nature talks on a wide variety of subjects. I have attended programs on wildlife spotting, big cats of the southwest, owls, native cutthroat trout, and wildfire prevention. It is a really worthwhile educational program, ideal for kids, and the interns make it fun.

GETTING THERE

From Jemez Falls Ranger Station, drive north on US 4 for 9.5 miles, and turn left into campground.

GPS COORDINATES

UTM Zone (WGS84) 13S
Easting 0353008
Northing 3969743
Latitude N 35° 51' 39.2"
Longtitude W 106° 37' 40.8"

15
JEMEZ FALLS
CAMPGROUND

> *The pride of the Jemez area*

LOCATED IN A VALLEY SURROUNDED by towering ponderosa pine and aspens, Jemez Falls Campground is the pride of the Jemez area. Jemez Falls is one of the newer campgrounds in the Jemez Wilderness, and it is sparkling clean. Tents and RVs cohabitate well at this campground, and pop-up campers and trailers are common. With many large campsites and generous spacing between sites, your time spent here will be peaceful. Of all the campgrounds in this book, this is the author's number one choice. Four loops exist within the campground, and the large RVs tend to prefer the loop to the far right. This loop is the closest to NM 4 and receives some highway noise. Due to the campground topography, and distance from the highway, highway noise is not a factor on the other loops. There are no reserveable sites at this campground.

Tent campers have many delightful spaces, and most spots are shady due to the dense canopy of ponderosas. Most campsites are quite grassy and level. You will notice outcroppings of young ponderosas throughout the campground. Forest thinning has not taken place here, so you will enjoy the forest's beauty. This campground is popular, so get here as early as possible if your outing is planned on a weekend. Even with a full campground, it's surprisingly quiet. Camping here during the week is phenomenal if you love serenity.

You will see plenty of blue jays, several species of woodpeckers, and a large population of hummingbirds. This is bear country, though, so read and adhere to the posted signs. Bobcat, mountain lion, and coyote are common carnivores here, but generally fight shy of this area. There have been a few reports of a large male coyote spotted in the campground. If you bring pets, keep them on a leash at all times and be wary. Deer and elk herds are common in this area, but

RATINGS

Beauty: ☆ ☆ ☆ ☆ ☆
Privacy: ☆ ☆ ☆ ☆
Spaciousness: ☆ ☆ ☆ ☆ ☆
Quiet: ☆ ☆ ☆ ☆
Security: ☆ ☆ ☆ ☆ ☆
Cleanliness: ☆ ☆ ☆ ☆ ☆

migrate to remote areas in the Santa Fe National Forest when camping season arrives. Be careful driving down NM 4 because wildlife cross this road frequently.

Four vault toilets are distributed conveniently and kept spotless. Jemez Falls has an underground pressurized well. Improvements were completed on the system in 2006, and brand-new water spigots have been added near each toilet. The water does have a trace of chlorine, so filtering is recommended.

Jemez Falls has an amphitheater, and it is used often by Forest Service interns who put on educational and entertaining nature programs most weekends. There is also a nondenominational church service held every Sunday morning at 8 a.m., and it is enjoyable and uplifting.

Kids love the campground, and there are plenty of places for them to play safely. The 1.5-mile road through the campground has a few hills, and it is an absolute blast on a bicycle. The speed limit is posted at 10 miles per hour and strictly enforced. U.S. Forest Service law enforcement and the Sandovol County Sheriff Department patrol this campground often, so you are safe here. There is a campground host on duty from Memorial Day through Labor Day.

Jemez Falls may be opened as early as the first weekend in May, but the water is never turned on until the host arrives. The campground is kept open until the end of September, but the Forest Service may close several loops as the crowds dwindle.

This campground has been picked clean of firewood, but several forest roads nearby have plenty of downed wood to gather. The campground host sells wood for $6 a bundle.

June 6, 2007, was a day that almost marked an end to this campground. After over a week without rain, a terrible fire raged out of control, and stopped within 50 feet of the campsites. The fire was apparently caused by heat lightning and jumped two fire lines before it was brought under control. The following Saturday afternoon, the rains came and soaked the lovely forest.

KEY INFORMATION

ADDRESS: Jemez Ranger District P.O. Box 150 Jemez Springs, NM 87025 (505) 829-3535 www.fs.fed.us/ r3/sfe

OPERATED BY: Santa Fe National Forest U.S. Department of Agriculture

OPEN: Opens early May, closes mid-September; official season Memorial Day–Labor Day

SITES: 52; all sites are first come, first served

EACH SITE HAS: Parking space, picnic table, and fire ring

REGISTRATION: Self-service registration, immediately upon selecting campsite

FEE: $10 per night single unit; $20 per night double unit

ELEVATION: 8,007 feet

RESTRICTIONS: *Pets:* On leash, 6-foot maximum
Fires: Wood fires permitted only in provided fire rings; charcoal grills are permitted
Alcohol: Within campsite only
Quiet Hours: 10 p.m.–8 a.m.
Stay Limit: 14 days

MAP

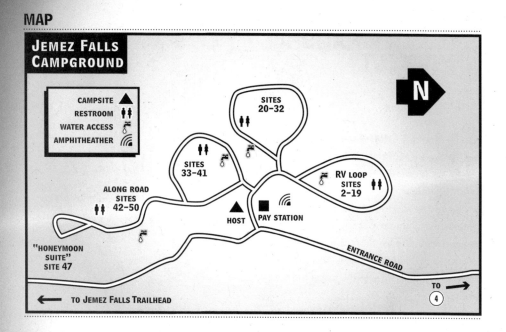

JEMEZ FALLS CAMPGROUND

CAMPSITE ▲
RESTROOM ♀♂
WATER ACCESS
AMPHITHEATHER

N

SITES 20-32

SITES 33-41

RV LOOP SITES 2-19

ALONG ROAD SITES 42-50

HOST   PAY STATION

"HONEYMOON SUITE" SITE 47

ENTRANCE ROAD

← TO JEMEZ FALLS TRAILHEAD

TO → 4

GETTING THERE

From Jemez Springs Ranger Station, drive north on NM 4 for 11.5 miles. Turn right at Jemez Falls Campground sign and follow road 1 mile to campground.

Outside of the campground to the south, the Jemez Falls Trail leads to the majestic waterfalls. The trail is 1 mile in length, an easy-to-moderate hike until you reach the end. The final descent to the falls is quite steep, so please exercise caution. At the end of the trail, a primitive log ladder provides access to the pool below the falls.

GPS COORDINATES

UTM Zone (WGS84) 13S
Easting 0354916
Northing 3965583
Latitude N 35° 49' 25.3"
Longtitude W 106° 36' 22.1"

16
BANDELIER NATIONAL MONUMENT

JUNIPER **C**AMPGROUND is an awesome place for a getaway and unique within the Jemez Wilderness area. This campground is operated by the National Park Service. The campground is atop a volcanic mesa, dotted with juniper, pinon, and ponderosa pine. Juniper Campground has 94 sites compressed within three loops, but some spots will afford you privacy. Some campsites lack shade. Hiking around the area, I gathered pinon nuts, a delightful camp snack.

I camped here in April of 2006 on the east loop at campsite 8. It was an ideal site, with a close water spigot, right across from the restrooms. This campsite has a large ponderosa that gave me nice shade, and some juniper bushes for privacy. The campsites are rocky, so bring adequate ground padding. There will be a few RVs, but this is a popular campground for tent campers, and it is quiet.

A picnic table and fire ring are provided at each campsite. Numerous campsites are handicap accessible. Three tents and two vehicles are allowed at each site. The restrooms are modern, with sinks and flush toilets, and are kept spotless. The water is treated with chlorine, so filtering is recommended.

A campground host is here between Memorial Day and Labor Day. Gathering firewood is prohibited, but the camp host sells bundles of firewood. National Park Service officers patrol this campground frequently, and you will be safe. Rules and policies are strictly adhered to, but the officers are friendly and helpful. An electronic self-pay station is located at the entrance of the loops; select your site first and then pay immediately.

This is bear country, so abide by posted precautions. You may spot mule deer, turkey, coyote, jackrabbit, chipmunks, and Abert's squirrels. In warm weather

> *Bandelier's human history dates back 10,000 years.*

RATINGS

Beauty: ☆ ☆ ☆ ☆
Privacy: ☆ ☆ ☆
Spaciousness: ☆ ☆ ☆
Quiet: ☆ ☆ ☆ ☆ ☆
Security: ☆ ☆ ☆ ☆ ☆
Cleanliness: ☆ ☆ ☆ ☆ ☆

KEY INFORMATION

ADDRESS: Bandelier National Monument
HCR 1, Box1
Los Alamos, NM 87544
(505) 672-3861
www.nps.gov/band/

OPERATED BY: Bandelier National Monument National Park Service

OPEN: Campground opening depends on weather; official season Memorial Day–Labor Day

SITES: 94; all sites are first come, first served

EACH SITE HAS: Parking space, picnic table, and fire ring

REGISTRATION: Self-service registration, immediately upon selecting campsite

FEES: 7-day automobile/vehicle permit $12; Bandelier National Monument Annual Pass $30; $12 per night single unit

ELEVATION: 6,672 feet at entrance

RESTRICTIONS: *Pets:* On leash, 6-foot maximum; pets are not allowed on any trails within the park; pets are allowed in the campground, picnic areas, and in parking areas only
Fires: Wood fires permitted only in provided fire rings: charcoal fires permitted in grills
Alcohol: Within campsite only
Quiet Hours: 10 p.m.–8 a.m.
Stay Limit: 14 days

you may spot rattlesnakes. There are several species here, including the western prairie rattlesnake and the western diamondback. Educate yourself regarding venomous reptiles, watch your children closely, and keep your pets leashed and under control.

Summers are quite hot here, reaching the upper 90s. Spring and fall are ideal seasons to visit, and the campground rarely fills up before Memorial Day or after Labor Day. Summer thunderstorms can be sudden and violent, so be ready to take evasive action. Spring weather is unpredictable, with cold nights until mid-May. Daytime temperatures in spring and fall are generally in the 50°F to 60°F range. Fall camping is pleasant here through mid-October. Because this campground sits atop a mesa, it can get quite windy.

More than 70 miles of hiking trails wind throughout the national monument. The most popular hike begins at the visitor center and leads to Frijoles Canyon. You will find several excavation sites and the "cavates," a network of human-carved caves in the cliffside. The main archeological sites were inhabited from the 1100s into the mid-1500s.

For those who love history and culture, Bandelier's human history dates back 10,000 years, when nomadic hunters followed game through the canyons. Ancestors of modern Pueblo people built thriving communities here 600 years ago. Remnants of several thousand dwellings have been found among the mesas and steep canyons.

At the visitor center there is a snack bar, a gift shop, and a well-stocked bookstore. Interpretive ranger-led hikes are a popular activity, as is the Bandelier Museum exhibit.

MAP

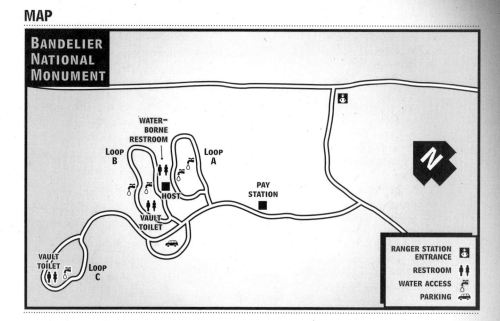

GETTING THERE

From Los Alamos, travel west on NM 4 for 11.5 miles, through the town of White Rock. The Bandelier Monument entrance is on the left side of the road.

GPS COORDINATES

UTM Zone (WGS84) 13S
Easting 0384734.2
Northing 3961649.1
Latitude N 35° 47' 31.84"
Longtitude W 106° 16' 31.95"

17
FENTON LAKE STATE PARK CAMPGROUND

> *Fenton Lake is loved by many who call this place home for the weekend.*

FENTON LAKE STATE PARK was one of the most beautiful state parks in New Mexico until the Lakes Fire of August 27, 2002. This fire was started by a camper and destroyed more than 4,000 acres, including the ridge to the south, known as Lake Fork Mesa. The fire damage can be viewed from anywhere in the park. The park was spared from the flames. The rains came just in time, dowsing the fire for the weary firefighters.

Fenton Lake is still a delightful state park; loved by many who continue to call this place home for the weekend. The campground itself remains beautiful, despite the surrounding areas devastated by the fire. The campground is set in a deep forest of ponderosa pines. The campground is active with Stellar's jays, various woodpeckers, and many hummingbirds. Bird-watchers spot raptors regularly here, including the peregrine falcon.

There is a large population of chipmunks, which love campers and can almost be fed by hand. Fenton Lake is home to several species of ducks and geese, turkey, mule deer, muskrat, elk, bobcat, mountain lion, and black bear.

This state park does a good job separating RVs from tent campers. Loops A, B, and C are day-use areas. Loop D is the RV loop and is large. A sign beyond loop D prohibits RVs from entering the other loops. Loops E and F are the areas we tent campers call home. Just a warning: the sites along the road are vulnerable to a cloud of fine dust every time a vehicle passes. The best sites are at the far end of the camp,

RATINGS*

Beauty: ☆ ☆ ☆ ☆ ☆
Privacy: ☆ ☆ ☆
Spaciousness: ☆ ☆ ☆
Quiet: ☆ ☆ ☆ ☆
Security: ☆ ☆ ☆ ☆ ☆
Cleanliness: ☆ ☆ ☆ ☆ ☆

*Note: Beauty rating was judged on campground, not on the nearby fire damage. Cleanliness does not take into account the road dust; the facilities are spotless.

away from traffic. The dusty road is the main drawback of camping at this park; asphalt roads and camping pads would be an asset here.

Each campsite comes equipped with a parking spot, a pedestal grill, a fire grate, and a picnic table. Two vehicles and two tents are allowed at each site. All campsites are fairly level and not too rocky. There are grassy areas to pitch your tent, but most campsites have a large dirt area. The area is being thinned of timber, yet most sites have excellent shade. There is a vault toilet located on each loop, plus a wheelchair-access toilet located near the wheelchair-accessible camping areas along the roadway. A children's playground lies near loop E. There are only two water spigots, one located at loop C and one at the parking area on the southwestern corner of the lake. The well is treated with chlorine, so filtering is recommended.

Annual precipitation averages 19 inches. Summer temperatures rise to around 80°F and can drop into the low 40s many nights. Winter temperatures range from daytime 30s and 40s to single digits in winter. This is one of few campgrounds in the mountains of New Mexico that stays open all winter. The lake is popular for ice fishing, cross-country skiing, and camping for hunters in early spring or fall.

The Fenton State Park rangers are friendly but strict, and the Sandovol County Sheriff's Department patrols with regularity. The New Mexico Fish and Game Department checks licenses and possession limits frequently.

The fishing here is excellent, and the lake and nearby streams are stocked regularly with rainbow trout by the Seven Springs fish hatchery 2 miles to the north on NM 126. You can visit the Seven Springs Fish Hatchery; admission is free, and there is a kid's fishing pond stocked with some large fish. The hatchery also breeds the Rio Grand cutthroat trout and the German brown trout.

Fenton Lake was built in 1946 when a dam was built on Cebolla Creek. The 35-acre lake features a cross-country ski and biathlon trail and wheelchair-accessible fishing platforms. The 2-mile Hal Baxter

KEY INFORMATION

ADDRESS: Fenton Lake State Park
455 Fenton Lake Road
Jemez Springs, NM 87025
(505) 829-3630
www.emnrd.state.nm.us/PRD/Fenton.htm

OPERATED BY: New Mexico State Parks Department

OPEN: Year-round

SITES: 40 individual sites; all sites are first come, first served

EACH SITE HAS: Parking space, picnic table, and fire ring

REGISTRATION: Self-service registration, immediately upon selecting campsite

FEE: $10 per night developed site; $4 electrical hook-up

ELEVATION: 7,654 feet

RESTRICTIONS: *Pets:* On leash, 6-foot maximum (strictly enforced); take precautionary measures for predators
Fires: Wood fires permitted only in provided fire rings; charcoal grills are permitted
Alcohol: Within campsite only
Quiet Hours: 10 p.m.–8 a.m.
Stay Limit: 14 days

MAP

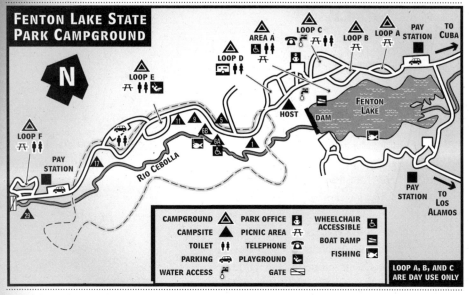

FENTON LAKE STATE PARK CAMPGROUND

N

LOOP C
AREA A
LOOP B
LOOP A
PAY STATION
TO CUBA
LOOP D
LOOP E
LOOP F
PAY STATION
HOST
DAM
FENTON LAKE
RIO CEBOLLA
PAY STATION
TO LOS ALAMOS

CAMPGROUND		PARK OFFICE	
CAMPSITE		PICNIC AREA	
TOILET		TELEPHONE	
PARKING		PLAYGROUND	
WATER ACCESS		GATE	

WHEELCHAIR ACCESSIBLE
BOAT RAMP
FISHING

LOOP A, B, AND C ARE DAY USE ONLY

GETTING THERE

From Jemez Springs, drive 11 miles to La Cueva, turn west (left) onto NM 126. Drive 11 miles to Fenton Lake and turn left at the sign.

Trail loops the park and provides opportunities to view wildlife in its natural habitat. The 135-acre lake provides excellent trout fishing. Float tubes, canoes, inflatable rafts, kayaks, and small fishing boats are welcome. Trolling motors are allowed.

GPS COORDINATES

UTM Zone (WGS84) 13S
Easting 0344332
Northing 3972629
Latitude 35° 53' 08.0"
Longtitude 106° 43' 28.6"

18
CLEAR CREEK
CAMPGROUND

I **N THE PRISTINE MOUNTAINS** above the town of Cuba, two pretty campgrounds 1 mile apart are a must-visit for the tent camper. Although smaller in size than the other Jemez Wilderness camps in this book, Clear Creek and Rio de las Vacas (see page 77) are for those who want more remote camping with the benefits of an established campground.

Clear Creek is the first campground you reach as you drive up NM 126 from Cuba. The road is now paved past Clear Creek. Previously the traffic along NM 126 would stir gigantic dust clouds that drifted into this camp. Both Clear Creek and Rio De Las Vacas campgrounds were closed during the 2003 and 2004 camping seasons for extensive renovations. The campground loops and parking pads have been paved. The asphalt is a welcome addition here, because the campground was previously dusty.

Brand-new wheelchair-accessible vault toilets have been added. All campsites are equipped with new pedestal grills, fire grates, and picnic tables. The water system is provided by a deep well and hand pump. The water should be filtered because the well is treated with chlorine.

Clear Creek has a tiny stream several inches deep and about a foot wide running through the heart of the campground. The cool water is ideal for foot soaking after a rugged hike. There are no pools to fish here, but it adds to the ambience of the place.

Clear Creek has a group-camping area set deep against a hill in the back of the campground. This area has a 40-foot-diameter gazebo and parking separated from the rest of the campground. The group site has capacity for 12 tents and can be reserved. Numerous pedestal grills and fire grates are available for the group area.

Clear Creek offers 12 individual campsites, and all

> *Remote camping with the benefits of an established campground.*

RATINGS

Beauty: ✿ ✿ ✿ ✿ ✿
Privacy: ✿ ✿ ✿ ✿
Spaciousness: ✿ ✿ ✿ ✿
Quiet: ✿ ✿ ✿ ✿ ✿
Security: ✿ ✿ ✿ ✿ ✿
Cleanliness: ✿ ✿ ✿ ✿ ✿

KEY INFORMATION

ADDRESS: Cuba Ranger
District
P.O. Box130
Cuba, NM 87103
(505) 289-3264
www.fs.fed.us/r3/sfe

OPERATED BY: Santa Fe National
Forest
U.S. Department of
Agriculture

OPEN: Official season,
Memorial Day–
Labor Day

SITES: 12 individual sites;
all sites are first
come, first served; 1
group site, up to 60
campers

EACH SITE HAS: Parking space, picnic
table, and fire ring

REGISTRATION: Self-service registration, immediately
upon selecting
campsite

FEE: $10 per night single
unit, maximum 2
vehicles per site; $10
per night for each
additional vehicle;
$50 per night group;
contact Cuba
Ranger District for
reservations

ELEVATION: 8,389 feet

RESTRICTIONS: *Pets:* On leash, 6-foot
maximum
Fires: Wood fires
permitted only in
provided fire rings;
charcoal grills are
permitted
Alcohol: Within
campsite only
Quiet Hours: 10 p.m.–
8 a.m.
Stay Limit: 14 days

are well spaced and private. Due to the past few years of rain, the grass has really filled in here, and tent camping is wonderful. There is no road noise, and quiet hours are respected. The campground is in a mixed coniferous forest, primarily of ponderosa pines, spruce, fir, and a few aspen trees. Most sites are shaded. Several sites are designated wheelchair accessible.

Clear Creek is open one week before Memorial Day through one week after Labor Day. Patrols are made by Santa Fe National Forest law enforcement officers and the Sandovol County Sheriff's Department. Forest Service employees are always working in this area, so the campground is safe. Cuba Ranger District generally assigns a host here to take care of both Clear Creek and Rio de las Vacas camps.

There is no cellular service at Clear Creek. The nearest cellular service is in Cuba, 11.4 miles away. Cuba has several stores with camping and fishing supplies. There is CC's Paisano Pizzeria, a good break from camp cooking, and a Frosty Freez for ice-cream addicts like myself.

Due to the remoteness of this campsite and the creek, black bears and other wildlife are common. Raccoons will wreak havoc. If you read and comply with the bear-alert signs that are posted, you will have no problems with any of the wildlife. Keep pets on a leash at all times and watch children closely. This campground is equipped with a cattle guard at the entrance, and the perimeter is fenced, so you will not wake up with a 2,000 pound Angus at your camp.

MAP

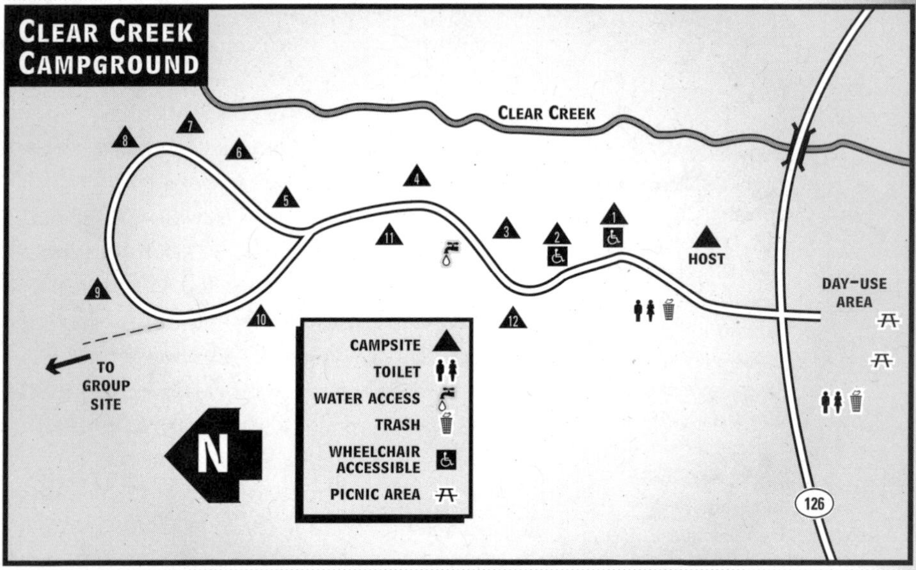
CLEAR CREEK CAMPGROUND
CLEAR CREEK
1
2
3
4
5
6
7
8
9
10
11
12
HOST
DAY-USE AREA
TO GROUP SITE
N
CAMPSITE
TOILET
WATER ACCESS
TRASH
WHEELCHAIR ACCESSIBLE
PICNIC AREA
126

GETTING THERE

From US 550 in Cuba, turn right at the small tourist office and follow NM for 126 11.4 miles; the campground will be on the left.

GPS COORDINATES

UTM Zone (WGS84) 13S
Easting 0335372.7
Northing 3985080.7
Latitude N 35° 59' 46.7"
Longtitude W 106° 49' 37.1"

19
RIO DE LAS VACAS CAMPGROUND

> *A rushing stream, cascading over boulders with several chest-deep pools, runs the length of the campground.*

THE NAME *RIO DE LAS VACAS* means "river of the cattle" in Spanish. This pretty camp is just 1 mile from Clear Creek campground. Warning: this is open-range country and cattle abound. You may see cowboys punching cattle along the road. Obey the cowboys' hand signals and instructions; in open range areas, livestock always have the right of way. Cattle cross this road frequently, so please drive carefully. When hiking, keep your distance from livestock. When walking along New Mexico 126, beware of traffic because four-wheel-drive vehicles, ATVs, and motorcycles speed frequently along this road.

This campground is somewhat larger than Clear Creek, and the campsites are more spacious. The first eight campsites you see to the right are along the stream. Arriving early is recommended if you want one of these spots, because these sites fill up first. The stream-side campsites may pose some inevitable intrusion; anglers may walk through your camp en route to the stream. The road then loops to the left and up a slight incline where the remaining campsites are found.

Rio de las Vacas offers 16 individual campsites, each equipped with a picnic table and fire ring. There is no road noise, and quiet hours are respected. The campground is in a mixed coniferous forest, with ponderosa pines, spruce, fir, and a few aspen trees. There are grassy areas to pitch your tent. Due to the forest canopy, most sites are shaded and are wheelchair accessible.

This campground was closed during the 2003 and 2004 camping seasons for renovation. Prior to 2005, the loops were repaired and are oiled gravel. Brand-new wheelchair-accessible vault toilets (the no-odor type), new fire grates, and picnic tables were added.

The water system is provided by a well and hand pump. The water is pure and sweet tasting, but filtering is advisable.

RATINGS

Beauty: ☆ ☆ ☆ ☆ ☆
Privacy: ☆ ☆ ☆ ☆
Spaciousness: ☆ ☆ ☆ ☆
Quiet: ☆ ☆ ☆ ☆ ☆
Security: ☆ ☆ ☆ ☆ ☆
Cleanliness: ☆ ☆ ☆ ☆ ☆

Rios de las Vacas opens one week prior to Memorial Day and closes one week after Labor Day. Santa Fe National Forest law enforcement officers and the Sandovol County Sheriff's Department patrol occasionally. Forest Service employees are always in this area, so security is good.

Rio de las Vacas is a rushing stream cascading over boulders and several chest-deep pools. In the spring snowmelt, this stream becomes a real torrent, so watch children closely while they play near it. The stream can be heard throughout the campground. During the monsoon season this stream can get dangerous when flash floods occur, so be ready. It is recommended to pitch your tent on the high ground, because this stream will overrun its banks.

Trout anglers have good success here. This stream starts at the head water of San Gregorio Lake. Anglers catch several species of trout in the stream: brook, brown, and rainbow. San Gregorio Lake is accessible 1 mile uphill from a marked trail in this campground, and the fishing is generally good.

As the stream makes its way under the bridge at NM 126, it meanders into an open meadow where you can find the ruins of an old cabin. This meadow is a lovely place to spend time, and it explodes in color with wildflowers throughout the summer.

There is no cellular service at the campground. The nearest cellular service and pay telephones are located in Cuba, 12.4 miles away. Cuba has several stores; Saveway Market and Variety Store, and a True Value Hardware Store. Both carry camping and fishing supplies and sell New Mexico state fishing licenses. There is also a CC's Paisano Pizzeria, and a Frosty Freez to tempt ice-cream addicts.

Due to the remoteness of this campsite and the creek, black bears have been spotted in the camp. Raccoons can cause problems here. If you read and comply with the bear-alert signs that are posted, you will have no problems with any of the wildlife. Keep pets on a leash at all times and watch children closely. There is a cattle guard at the entrance, and the perimeter is fenced, so cattle will not intrude.

KEY INFORMATION

ADDRESS: Cuba Ranger District P.O. Box130 Cuba, NM 87103 (505) 289-3264 www.fs.fed.us/r3/sfe

OPERATED BY: Santa Fe National Forest U.S. Department of Agriculture

OPEN: Official season, Memorial Day–Labor Day

SITES: 16 individual sites; all sites are first come, first served

EACH SITE HAS: Parking space, picnic table, and fire ring

REGISTRATION: Self-service registration, immediately upon selecting campsite

FEE: $10 per night single unit

ELEVATION: 7,880 feet

RESTRICTIONS: *Pets:* On leash, 6-foot maximum
Fires: Wood fires permitted only in provided fire rings; charcoal grills are permitted
Alcohol: Within campsite only
Quiet Hours: 10 p.m.–8 a.m.
Stay Limit: 14 days

MAP

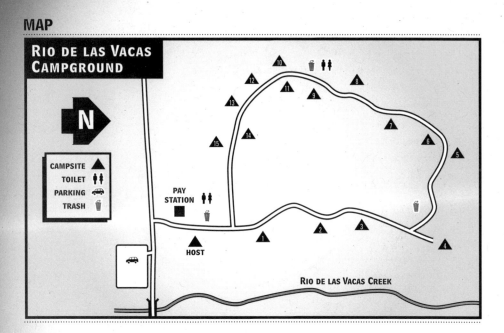

RIO DE LAS VACAS CAMPGROUND

N

CAMPSITE ▲
TOILET 🚹🚺
PARKING 🚗
TRASH 🗑

PAY STATION 🚹🚺

HOST ▲

RIO DE LAS VACAS CREEK

GETTING THERE

From US 550 in Cuba, turn right at the small tourist office and follow NM 126 12.4 miles; the campground will be on the left.

GPS COORDINATES

UTM Zone (WGS84) 13S
Easting 0337153.2
Northing 3985075.8
Latitude N 35° 59' 47.61"
Longtitude W 106° 48' 24.03"

NORTH CENTRAL CAMPGROUNDS:
SANTA FE NATIONAL FOREST
Santa Fe, Pecos, Las Vegas Area

20
BLACK CANYON
CAMPGROUND

> *A deep canyon filled with ponderosa pine, blue spruce, fir, aspen, and cottonwoods*

SANTA FE HAS SOME REALLY pretty campgrounds nearby, and the newest is Black Canyon Campground. Black Canyon is 7.5 miles from downtown Santa Fe, and the drive there is gorgeous. A winding road works its way from high desert yucca- and sage-filled hills to a deep lush green canyon filled with ponderosa pine, blue spruce, fir, aspen, and tall cottonwood trees.

The Black Canyon is so named because the canyon is steep and deep. While Santa Fe is waking to the early morning rays of sunlight, the canyon remains dark until the sun crests over the mountain. While the city basks in its sunlight at dawn, the canyon darkens an entire hour before the sun goes down—wonderful for campers who want a few extra winks of sleep.

The entrance to Black Canyon is on the right side of the road. As you enter the campground, you'll find everything new and sparkling clean. The campground was renovated in 2006. There is a parking lot for the adjoining day-use area, which contains a large gazebo and plenty of space for picnics and other large events. The entrance also houses modern vault toilets and a water spigot whose source is from Santa Fe city water supply.

The tent sites begin at the entrance and are adjacent to the highway, which is prone to road noise. One large wheelchair-accessible tent site is separated from five other tent sites. These sites are walk-in, and the pathways are asphalt. Another water spigot and varmint-proof trash receptacle are located halfway down the path. Each of these tent sites is separated by low shrubbery and shaded by the tall conifer forest. A small intermittent stream runs parallel to the path. The tent sites are spaced apart fairly well.

The road runs up the hill past the campground host's space, and all drive-in sites are compacted tightly.

RATINGS

Beauty: ✿ ✿ ✿ ✿ ✿
Privacy: ✿
Spaciousness: ✿
Quiet: ✿ ✿ ✿
Security: ✿ ✿ ✿ ✿ ✿
Cleanliness: ✿ ✿ ✿ ✿ ✿

Beginning at site 7, all sites are equipped with a concrete pad, a gravel tent area, fire ring, lantern pole, and picnic table. Although several sites are designated for wheelchairs, all sites would be accommodating. A total of five wheelchair-accessible toilet buildings, each with a water spigot and trash receptacle, are spread conveniently around the loop. Two commercial-size dumpsters are located in the camp. There is no firewood available here, but you can drive up NM 475 toward the Santa Fe Ski Basin and find plenty of fallen aspen branches alongside the road, or bring your own.

The camp is beautiful and peaceful in appearance. The rockwork and terracing are designed well. If the sites were further spaced, this would be a five-star campground. It is apparent that the architect hasn't spent much time tent camping.

For the solitude of all who come here, this campground has adopted a new policy regarding generator use. Generators are allowed to be run for 30 minutes every three hours. Good policy, but enforcing it is another matter.

The campground opens in April and closes at the end of October. Spring, fall, and weekdays are ideal times to camp here with peace and quiet, avoiding the crowds.

Sites 23, 26, and 27 are double sites, and are $20 per night. Security is excellent; a host is assigned here, the Forest Service patrols frequently, and the Santa Fe County Sheriff's Department stops by. A 1-mile hiking trail circles the perimeter of the camp, accessible from the back of the camp.

KEY INFORMATION

ADDRESS: Espanola Ranger District
P.O. Box 3307
Espanola, NM 87113
(505) 753-7331
www.fs.fed.us/r3/sfe

OPERATED BY: Espanola Ranger District, Santa Fe National Forest U.S. Department of Agriculture

OPEN: April 1–November 1, weather permitting

SITES: 36 sites; reservations accepted online at www.recreation.gov; other sites first come, first served

EACH SITE HAS: Parking space, picnic table, lantern hanger, and fire ring

REGISTRATION: Self-service registration, immediately upon selecting campsite

FEE: $10 per night single unit

ELEVATION: 8,323 feet

RESTRICTIONS: *Pets:* On leash, 6-foot maximum; take precautionary measures for predators; bear and mountain lion have been spotted
Fires: Wood fires in fire rings only; charcoal grills are permitted
Alcohol: At campsite
Quiet Hours: 10 p.m.–8 a.m.
Stay Limit: 14 days

MAP

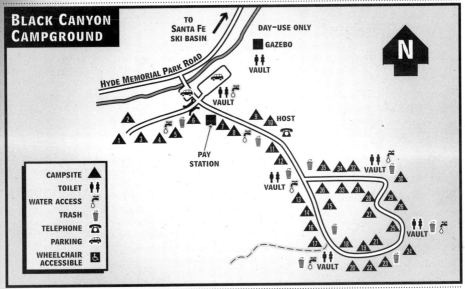

GETTING THERE

Take Bishop's Lodge Road to
Artist Road, which will turn
into NM 475, also known as
Hyde Park Road, and travel
7.5 miles to the campground.

GPS COORDINATES

UTM Zone (WGS84) 13S
Easting 0424036
Northing 3954113
Latitude 35° 43' 41.0"
Longtitude 105° 50' 23.9"

21
FIELD TRACT CAMPGROUND

I F YOU WANT A LITTLE SLICE of heaven, Field Tract Campground is a great choice. This camp is easy to get to, located off NM 63, just a scant 10 miles north of the historic little town of Pecos. Field Tract is the first developed campground you will come to after entering the Pecos River Wilderness. The Pecos River runs past this campground at a thundering pace, cascading over boulders and filling the entire campground with its lovely music. Although located along NM 63, this campground is peaceful, and the river drowns out the road noise nicely at most campsites.

Bob, the campground host I met in 2007, served at this campground for 15 years. He is from Texas and the kindest gentleman you will ever meet. He keeps the place spotless and makes you wish there wasn't a stay limit. He is a textbook example of a perfect host. Bob sells firewood for $5 a bundle, but any nearby forest road will provide gathering spots for all the wood you need.

Field Tract is a large one-loop campground, with 15 campsites. Six of the sites, equipped with Adirondack shelters, are spread throughout the camp. The three-sided shelters are constructed of log and have rock fireplaces. The other campsites are each equipped with a picnic table and fire ring. The tall ponderosa pine trees provide lots of shade, with tall cottonwood trees skirting the river. The campground abounds in tall native grasses, almost eliminating the need for a ground pad in many areas.

Kids love this campground and have a safe place to pedal bicycles and ride scooters. Bird-watchers love this campground as do photographers. You are welcome to sit by Bob's birdfeeders and enjoy the many species that inhabit this forest. Hummingbirds are thick here and will entertain you for hours, so bring your

> *The Pecos River fills the entire campground with its lovely music.*

RATINGS

Beauty: ✩ ✩ ✩ ✩ ✩
Privacy: ✩ ✩ ✩ ✩
Spaciousness: ✩ ✩ ✩
Quiet: ✩ ✩ ✩ ✩ ✩
Security: ✩ ✩ ✩ ✩ ✩
Cleanliness: ✩ ✩ ✩ ✩ ✩

ADDRESS: Pecos Ranger
District
18 Highway 63
Pecos, NM 87552
(505) 757-6121
www.fs.fed.us/r3/sfe
/recreation/dis-
tricts/
pecos/index.html

OPERATED BY: Pecos Ranger
District
Santa Fe National
Forest
U.S. Department
of Agriculture

OPEN: Official season,
May 1–October 31

SITES: 15 individual sites;
all sites are first
come, first served

EACH SITE HAS: Parking space, picnic table, and fire
ring;
6 spaces with
Adirondack shelters

REGISTRATION: Self-service
registration,
immediately upon
selecting campsite

FEE: $10 per night single
unit

ELEVATION: 7,429 feet

RESTRICTIONS: *Pets:* On leash, 6-foot
maximum; take
precautionary
measures for
predators
Fires: Wood fires
permitted only in
provided fire rings;
charcoal grills are
permitted
Alcohol: Within
campsite only
Quiet Hours: 10 p.m.–
8 a.m.
Stay Limit: 14 days

feeder. Predators live in the area. Although no bears have been spotted at the campground lately, keep a wary eye just in case. On a starlit night in May, I was startled by one of two German shepherds who run loose in the camp, belonging to a nearby resident. They are shy and will cause you no trouble. Raccoons are plentiful here and will steal you blind, so pack away your food at night.

In the center of the campground is a large restroom, equipped with sinks and flush toilets. Two other vault toilets are located on the center loop between campsites 9 and 11. The center of the campground is grassy and shaded. The campsites are not the largest, but there is plenty of space between the sites. All campsites are level. Three pressurized water spigots are conveniently located across from site 1, between site 10 and 12, and in the center of the loop by the restroom.

Sites 7, 8, 10, and 12 are riverside campsites. Anglers must pass through these sites to access the river. The fishing here is good; the Pecos River is stocked with rainbow trout regularly by the New Mexico Game and Fish Department, which has numerous fish hatcheries throughout the state.

Security here is excellent; San Miguel County Sheriff's Department, U.S. Forest Service law enforcement officers, and New Mexico Game Wardens patrol this area constantly. Have your fishing license available because the fishing laws here are strictly enforced.

MAP

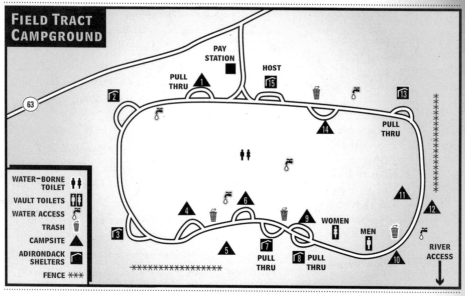

FIELD TRACT CAMPGROUND

PAY STATION

HOST

PULL THRU

63

WATER-BORNE TOILET
VAULT TOILETS
WATER ACCESS
TRASH
CAMPSITE
ADIRONDACK SHELTERS
FENCE ***

PULL THRU

WOMEN

MEN

RIVER ACCESS

PULL THRU

PULL THRU

GETTING THERE

From Pecos travel 10 miles north on NM 63, and the campground is on the right.

GPS COORDINATES

UTM Zone (WGS84) 13S
Easting 0437175
Northing 3949493
Latitude 35° 41' 14.4"
Longtitude 105° 41' 39.6"

> *Remote and somewhat secluded . . . a magnificent environment*

HOLY GHOST CAMPGROUND has been a popular campground in the Pecos Wilderness for many years. Remote and somewhat secluded, this campround is named for the Holy Ghost Creek that flows along its length. Despite its age, the campground has been updated with paved roads, which cut down on the dust. The environment is magnificent, where tall ponderosa pine, fir, spruce, aspen, and cottonwood trees make the shady campground appealing and restful. But this campground is busy.

Tent camping is popular here because of the grassy areas, but you will see a few RVs. The campsites are well spaced and reasonably large. After crossing the bridge into the campground, the road meanders back and forth to the end loop for 0.33 miles. Beyond the loop, an access road leads to a group camp, which if not reserved, serves as an overflow area. There are RVs at this campground. Generator usage is restricted to 30 minutes every three hours; however, it is unenforceable.

There are 25 campsites here on both sides of the road. The water is of questionable quality here; I pumped continuously and got a brown discoloration in the water samples I collected. It is recommended that you bring potable water. The loop has a parking area, and many backpackers launch off into the wilderness at the trailhead located here.

The streamside campsites are more appealing and provide the most shade. Three vault toilets are conveniently spaced throughout the camp The vault toilets are old and poorly vented. Most sites provide good grass for tents. Each site has a picnic table and fire ring, and varmint-proof trash receptacles are located near each toilet building. When the trash receptacles get full, the unwritten policy is to pack out your own trash.

RATINGS

Beauty: ✩ ✩ ✩ ✩
Privacy: ✩ ✩ ✩ ✩
Spaciousness: ✩ ✩ ✩ ✩ ✩
Quiet: ✩ ✩ ✩ ✩
Security: ✩ ✩ ✩
Cleanliness: ✩ ✩

Fishing is good along the creek, and anglers pull out some surprisingly large trout. Frequent visits by the New Mexico Game Wardens enforce stringent fishing laws and ensure camper's security. The U.S. Forest Service law enforcement patrols this campground regularly. There was no campground host assigned here in 2007.

The roadside is filled with lovely wildflowers, and many birds abound. Raccoons are frequent visitors, as are black bear. Rare visits by mountain lion and bobcat may occur at anytime, so be on guard. Elk are occasionally seen here, as are mule deer. Coyote inhabit this area; they are rarely seen but often heard at night.

Due to the elevation, summer daytime temperatures rarely exceed 85°F, and the nights can cool off into the 40s. Summer rains bring flash flooding along this creek, so be sure to wisely set up your tent away from the stream. There is plenty of firewood to gather in this area.

KEY INFORMATION

ADDRESS: Pecos Ranger District
18 Highway 63
Pecos, NM 87552
(505) 757-6121
www.fs.fed.us/r3/ sfe/recreation/ districts/pecos/ index.html

OPERATED BY: Pecos Ranger District
Santa Fe National Forest
U.S. Department of Agriculture

OPEN: Official season, mid-May– November 15, weather permitting

SITES: 25 individual sites; all sites are first come, first served

EACH SITE HAS: Parking space, picnic table, and fire ring

REGISTRATION: Self-service registration, immediately upon selecting campsite

FEE: $8 per night single unit

ELEVATION: 8,137 feet

RESTRICTIONS: *Pets:* On leash, 6-foot maximum; take precautionary measures for predators
Fires: Grills are permitted
Alcohol: Within campsite only
Quiet Hours: 10 p.m.–8 a.m.
Stay Limit: 14 days

MAP

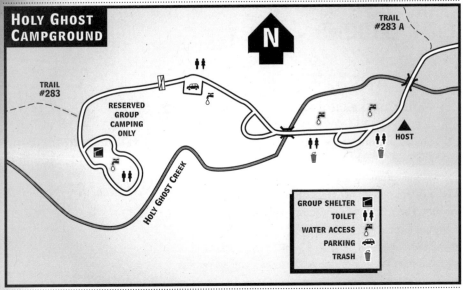

HOLY GHOST CAMPGROUND

TRAIL #283 A

TRAIL #283

RESERVED GROUP CAMPING ONLY

HOLY GHOST CREEK

HOST

GROUP SHELTER
TOILET
WATER ACCESS
PARKING
TRASH

GETTING THERE

From Pecos, drive 13.4 miles to Forest Service 122, which forks to the left. Follow FS 122 2.2 miles to the camp.

GPS COORDINATES

UTM Zone (WGS84) 13S
Easting 0436804
Northing 3958492
Latitude 35 46' 06.4"
Longtitude 105° 41' 56.9"

23
IRON GATE CAMPGROUND

IF YOU CAN ENDURE the gut-wrenching drive of 4.3 miles up Pecos' Forest Service 223, you will enjoy the camping experience of Iron Gate Campground. FS 223 is a four-wheel-drive road, not for the faint of heart. It takes about 20 minutes to get to the camp, potentially via a slippery mud bog when it rains. The road twists and turns with several steep hills and large rocks in the road. Do not attempt the drive without a high-clearance vehicle.

On my visit, Pecos Ranger District teams were out on a search and rescue training exercise, and several horse trailers were parked at the entrance of the camp. Despite their ability to get a horse trailer up to this camp, it would be unwise to attempt this road with an RV. I have not seen RVs here.

This lovely campground sits on a mountainside of Edelmann spruce, blue spruce, fir, and aspen. This is a one-loop campground, with good spacing between sites, and all the shaded sites are fairly private. Campsites 7 and 8 at the end of the loop are walk-in sites, less than 50 feet from the road. Campsites 1, 3, 11, 12, 13, and 14 are in the open with no shade, but the remaining sites are under the tree cover. The entire camp has deep grass, with wildflowers blooming. There are four horse corrals. One vault toilet is located at the entrance, and a second is located off the end loop. Two varmint-proof trash receptacles are located near the toilets. If the receptacles are full, you must pack out your trash.

There is no water, so pack in enough to douse your fire completely. An axe and shovel are mandatory at these remote camps, and I recommend a lawn rake as well. There is plenty of firewood along the road outside of the camp, especially downed aspen trees. If aspen wood is dry, it makes an excellent campfire.

There is plenty of parking, and the camp is graveled road. There isn't much traffic, so for the most

> *On a mountainside of edelman spruce, blue spruce, fir, and aspen*

RATINGS

Beauty: ✪ ✪ ✪ ✪ ✪
Privacy: ✪ ✪ ✪ ✪
Spaciousness: ✪ ✪ ✪ ✪ ✪
Quiet: ✪ ✪ ✪ ✪ ✪
Security: ✪ ✪
Cleanliness: ✪ ✪ ✪ ✪ ✪

ADDRESS: **Pecos Ranger District
18 Highway 63
Pecos, NM 87552
(505) 757-6121
www.fs.fed.us/r3/sfe/
recreation/districts/
pecos/index.html**

OPERATED BY: **Pecos Ranger District
Santa Fe National Forest
U.S. Department of Agriculture**

OPEN: **May 1–November 1, weather permitting**

SITES: **14 individual sites; all sites are first come, first served**

EACH SITE HAS: **Parking space, picnic table, and fire ring.**

REGISTRATION: **Self-service registration, immediately upon selecting campsite**

FEE: **$4 per night single unit**

ELEVATION: **9,243 feet**

RESTRICTIONS: *Pets:* **On leash, 6-foot maximum; take precautionary measures for predators**
Fires: **Wood fires permitted only in provided fire rings; charcoal grills are permitted**
Alcohol: **Within campsite only**
Quiet Hours: **10 p.m.– 8 a.m.**
Stay Limit: **14 days**

part, your camping will not be dusty. This camp is extremely clean thanks to conscientious campers. There is no host, but the Forest Service keeps an eye on this place. Due to its remoteness, predatory animals can frequent this camp. Please camp with this in mind.

This campground is high in elevation at over 9,200 feet, and it gets quite cold here overnight, so be sure to pack a warm sleeping bag. Expect lows in the low 40°F range nearly every night, even in the summer. Daytime temperatures will rarely exceed 80°F. When it rains, the runoff is good, but stake your tent on high ground. Bring a tarp to stretch over the picnic table. High elevations here in the Pecos Wilderness are susceptible to torrential downpours. Being on the side of a mountain poses issues with lightning strikes as well, so be ready to take cover.

Trailhead #250 begins at the end of the loop, is moderate to difficult, and travels a distance of 10 miles over elevations ranging from 9,200 to 11,400 feet. This trail is shared with horses. The trail usage is rated as light to moderately used.

MAP

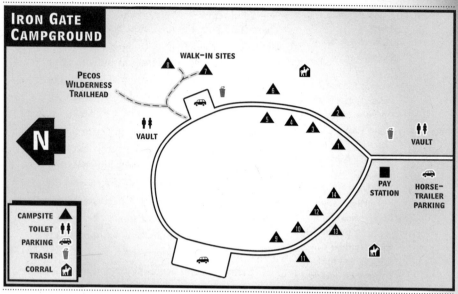

IRON GATE CAMPGROUND

WALK-IN SITES

PECOS WILDERNESS TRAILHEAD

VAULT

VAULT

PAY STATION

HORSE-TRAILER PARKING

CAMPSITE
TOILET
PARKING
TRASH
CORRAL

GETTING THERE

From Cowels, drive 0.75 miles south on NM 63 to FS 223. The road is well marked, so follow signs to campground. Drive slowly due to dust, and respect the homeowners along this road. Do not trespass on private property.

GPS COORDINATES

UTM Zone 13S
Easting 0443855
Northing 3966286
Latitude 35° 50' 20.9"
Longtitude 105° 37' 18.1

> *Worthy of a five-star rating*

IF THERE IS A CAMPGROUND worthy of a five-star rating, Jack's Creek has to be it. This campground is an absolute diamond. Jack's Creek is the last campground you come to in the Pecos Wilderness. Jack's Creek is second highest in elevation of the Pecos campgrounds at almost 9,000 feet. During my visit in late June, I heard woodpeckers working in the forests.

Surrounded in a lush grassy forest of tall, mature aspens, ponderosa, fir, and spruce trees, you would have to travel far to find a prettier location. The mountain vistas are breathtaking, with deep lush forests surrounding you by 360 degrees. The 12,622-foot Santa Fe Baldy is visible from the camp, with snowfields visible above tree line elevations well into July.

Jack's Creek is easily accessible, with paved roads all the way to the campground. The road hairpins and gets steep; there are no guardrails, and the road is not for the driver who fears heights. The camp is separated into three distinct areas; the equestrian camp, two group camps, and the main camping area. The equestrian camp is separated from the main camp by its own road. The two group camps, Group A and Group B, are by reservation only and cost $50 per night.

The campsites here are extremely large and well spaced for privacy. The sites on the inside of the loop have little shade but better grass. The campgrounds located on the outer loops have tall shady conifer and aspens but lack grass. All sites are level.

All restrooms are wheelchair accessible, equipped with composting toilets, and kept sparkling clean. A water spigot and trash receptacle are located at each restroom with other water spigots and trash receptacles placed at convenient locations around the camp. The water is clean and sweet tasting, but filtering is recommended.

RATINGS

Beauty: ✪ ✪ ✪ ✪ ✪
Privacy: ✪ ✪ ✪ ✪
Spaciousness: ✪ ✪ ✪ ✪ ✪
Quiet: ✪ ✪ ✪ ✪ ✪
Security: ✪ ✪ ✪ ✪ ✪
Cleanliness: ✪ ✪ ✪ ✪ ✪

The campground is secure, and a host is assigned here. Frequent patrols are made by the Forest Service, and the equestrian campground is a staging area for search and rescue operations.

All campsites come with a fire ring, picnic table, and gravel parking pad. All campsites accommodate tents as well as RVs. The campground is tent-camper friendly. Generator run times are restricted to 30 minutes every three hours and stay off at dark.

KEY INFORMATION

ADDRESS: Pecos Ranger District
18 Highway 63
Pecos, NM 87552
(505) 757-6121
www.fs.fed.us/r3/sfe/recreation/districts/pecos/index.html

OPERATED BY: Pecos Ranger District, Santa Fe National Forest U.S. Department of Agriculture

OPEN: Official season, Memorial Day–Labor Day

SITES: 39 sites; all first come, first served. 7 equestrian sites are first come, first served; some equestrian groups may reserve a site through the Pecos Ranger District

EACH SITE HAS: Parking space, picnic table, and fire ring.

REGISTRATION: Self-service registration upon selecting campsite

FEE: $10 per night single unit

ELEVATION: 8,936 feet

RESTRICTIONS: *Pets:* On leash, 6-foot maximum; take precautionary measures for predators
Fires: Wood fires only in provided fire rings; charcoal grills are permitted
Alcohol: Within campsite only
Quiet Hours: 10 p.m.–8 a.m.
Stay Limit: 14 days

MAP

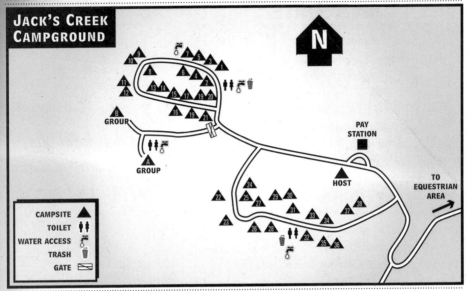

JACK'S CREEK CAMPGROUND

Legend:
- CAMPSITE ▲
- TOILET
- WATER ACCESS
- TRASH
- GATE

PAY STATION

HOST

TO EQUESTRIAN AREA

GROUP B

GROUP A

GETTING THERE

Follow NM 63 to Cowles; at the junction, follow Forest Service 555 for 3.4 miles to the campground.

GPS COORDINATES

UTM Zone (WGS84) 13S
Easting 35° 50' 19.1"
Northing 105° 39' 19.0"
Latitude 0440821
Longtitude 3966249

VILLANUEVA STATE PARK CAMPGROUND

SITUATED IN A LUSH FERTILE VALLEY, surrounded by mountains, mesas, and sheer dramatic cliffs, Villenueva Sate Park is a delightful place with the word *mañana* written all over it. The pace here is slow and relaxed, and takes you back to the 1800s. The park was named after the town of Villanueva you will pass through on your way to the park.

> *A delightful place with the word "mañana" written all over it.*

Villanueva State Park can be accessed from two separate directions. Coming from Santa Fe or Las Vegas, New Mexico, Villanueva is 12 miles south of the Interstate 25 exit. Driving from Albuquerque, the drive from I-40 north on NM 3 is the most scenic, as you make the breathtaking descent into this pretty, green valley. The name *Villenueva* means "new village" in Spanish; the town was established in 1890. Several old buildings and crumbling adobes seem to contradict the town's name. Two small general stores provide basic groceries but no camping supplies. The zip code directory of the entire valley lists only 217 addresses.

Villanueva State Park was established in 1967 and is one of the most modern facilities in the New Mexico park system. The park receives more than 48,000 visitors per year, and the majority of campers arrive over the weekends between May and September.

The park itself is set in a canyon of 500-foot-high red-and-yellow sandstone cliffs. With plenty of trees, you will have no trouble finding shade. The canyon walls block the sun in the mornings and afternoons. The campground altitude averages 5,800 feet, and it gets quite chilly in early spring or late fall. In the summer, the shady canyon is cooler than the open valley, where temperatures reach the high 90s.

Villanueva is open year-round; the gates are open from 7 a.m. to 7 p.m. every day from November through March. From April through September, the

RATINGS

Beauty: ☆ ☆ ☆ ☆ ☆
Privacy: ☆ ☆ ☆ ☆
Spaciousness: ☆ ☆ ☆ ☆
Quiet: ☆ ☆ ☆ ☆
Security: ☆ ☆ ☆ ☆ ☆
Cleanliness: ☆ ☆ ☆ ☆ ☆

KEY INFORMATION

ADDRESS: Villanueva State Park
P.O. Box 40
Villanueva, NM 87583
(505) 421-2957
www.emnrd.state
.nm.us/PRD/
Villanueva.htm

OPERATED BY: New Mexico State Parks

OPEN: Year-round

SITES: 33 individual sites; all sites are first come, first served

EACH SITE HAS: Parking space, picnic table, and fire ring

REGISTRATION: Self-service registration, immediately upon selecting campsite

FEE: $10 per night single unit; $4 electrical fee

ELEVATION: 5,749 feet

RESTRICTIONS: *Pets:* on leash, 6-foot maximum; take precautionary measures for predators
Fires: Wood fires permitted only in provided fire rings; charcoal grills are permitted
Alcohol: Within campsite only
Quiet Hours: 10 p.m.–8 a.m.
Stay Limit: 14 days

gate hours are from 7 a.m. until 9 p.m. every day. The rangers are helpful and friendly, and the park manager has been here for 21 years. They patrol often, as does the San Miguel County Sheriff's Department. The visitor center offers valuable information and several wildlife displays.

The campground is divided into several areas; the RV area is separated from the nonpowered campsites. Several tent sites are along the road at the park entrance, but they are small and afford no privacy. These campsites have adequate shade and a modern vault toilet with a water spigot. Across from these sites is the self-pay station.

Across from the pay station at the entrance are several small tent sites right along the road. These campsites have adequate shade, a modern vault toilet, and a water spigot.

The RV area is across the road from the visitor center. A large group picnic area and the comfort stations are located here. The comfort stations are equipped with showers and are spotlessly clean.

Past the group picnic shelter to the right are campsites located on both sides of the road. The best campsites are to the right, alongside the Pecos River. The soil at these riverside sites is a mix of sand and sparse grasses, making it a good choice for tent camping. The riverside area is quite shady, with a mix of Rio Grande cottonwood, coyote willow, Chinese elm, and mature juniper and pinon trees. These trees do a nice job of curtaining you from other campsites, and you will appreciate the privacy. Each of the campsites along the river has a covered shelter.

El Cerro camping area is up the hill and to the left; it holds ten campsites with several shelters and one modern vault toilet. The ground is quite rocky here, so bring a thick ground pad. Although you will not have the ambience of a riverside campground, you will be up on a hill with a great view of most of the park, the river, and the cliff sides.

Past the riverside campsites, there is a large picnic area and a modern playground. Children love Villanueva because there are safe places to play and nice areas for bicycle rides. The Pecos River runs year-

MAP

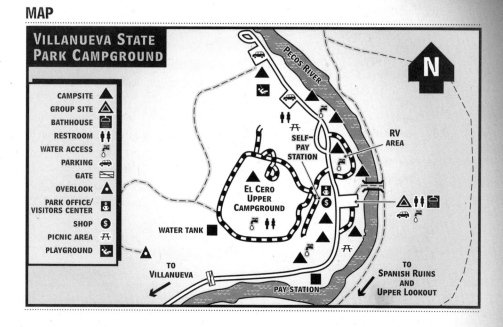

VILLANUEVA STATE PARK CAMPGROUND

Legend	
CAMPSITE	▲
GROUP SITE	△
BATHHOUSE	🛁
RESTROOM	🏻
WATER ACCESS	💧
PARKING	🚗
GATE	✉
OVERLOOK	▲
PARK OFFICE/VISITORS CENTER	📖
SHOP	$
PICNIC AREA	🏕
PLAYGROUND	🛝

PECOS RIVER

SELF-PAY STATION

RV AREA

EL CERO UPPER CAMPGROUND

WATER TANK ■

TO VILLANUEVA

PAY STATION

TO SPANISH RUINS AND UPPER LOOKOUT

N

round, and has a strong current during the spring snowmelt or during the monsoon season. Canoeing, tubing, rafting, and swimming are popular summer activities, but there is no lifeguard on duty. Before getting into the river, check with a ranger for any hazards you may encounter, and by all means be careful.

Coyote and black bear are common predators in the area, but tend to shy away when the crowds arrive in the summer. Be on the lookout for rattlesnakes; the western diamondback, and the prairie rattlesnake are indigenous in the park, so keep your pets reined in.

GETTING THERE

From Santa Fe:
Take I-25 Exit 363, follow NM 3 south for 12 miles through town of Villanueva, and follow sign to park.

From Albuquerque:
Take I-40 Exit 230, follow NM 3 north for 20 miles through town of Villanueva, and follow signs to park.

GPS COORDINATES

UTM Zone (WGS84) 13S
Easting 0469063
Northing 3902362
Latitude 35° 15' 50"
Longtitude 105° 20' 25"

> *Ideal desert-lake
> camping experience*

THE COCHITI LAKE CAMPGROUNDS offer ideal desert-lake camping experiences for many reasons. Cochiti dam is the 11th largest in the United States, using 65 million cubic feet of earth and rock. Construction took 10 years and was completed in 1975 at a cost of $94.4 million. There are two campgrounds, the main campground at Cochiti Lake headquarters, and Tetilla Peak Campground on the opposite side of the lake.

The main campground is open year-round; the Tetilla Peak Campground opens March 1 through October 31. Shoreline camping is not available at either campground.

The main Cochiti campground is divided into three loops, Loops A, B, and C. Loops B and C are designed for tent camping, while loop A is reserved for RVs.

Loop B, Chamisa Campground, has 34 campsites with 17 covered shelters. Lots of parking is available. There are two modern vault toilets in Juniper, at opposite ends of the loop. The waterborne restroom with the shower is a short walk up the hill from site 4. All restrooms are spotless. Due to juniper trees, bushes, and pinon trees, the campsites are semi-private.

Loop C, Apache Plume Campground, has 21 campsites with covered shelter, picnic table, and pedestal grill at each site. No restrooms or water spigots are available within this loop. This loop stays closed unless by group reservation or as an overflow area.

Loop A, Juniper Campground is the RV area. Each site has a water spigot and 30 or 50 ampere electrical hookups. Chamisa has three restrooms, and one is equipped with a shower.

Tetilla Peak Campground is divided into two loops for RVs with a total of 39 campsites and a small area for tents with 10 sites. There are three restrooms with

RATINGS

Beauty: ✿ ✿ ✿
Privacy: ✿ ✿
Spaciousness: ✿ ✿
Quiet: ✿ ✿ ✿ ✿ ✿
Security: ✿ ✿ ✿ ✿ ✿
Cleanliness: ✿ ✿ ✿ ✿ ✿

KEY INFORMATION

ADDRESS: Cochiti Lake Office
82 Dam Crest Road
Pena Blanca, NM 87041
(505)465-0307
www.spa.usace.army.mil/recreation/cochiti

OPERATED BY: United States Army Corps of Engineers, Albuquerque District

OPEN: Main campground open year-round; Tetilla Peak Campground open
April 1–October 31

SITES: Main campground, 77 individual sites; Tetilla Peak Campground, 52 individual sites; most sites reserved at www.recreation.gov or toll-free (877) 444-6777; if not reserved, sites are on a first-come, first-serve basis; inquire at main campground gate office for availability

EACH SITE HAS: Parking space, picnic table, and pedestal charcoal grill; many have covered shelters

REGISTRATION: Check in the office at campground entrance for registration; if office is unattended, self-registration is required

FEE: $8 per night, family tent site (max. 2 tents and 1 vehicle per site);
$12 per night, full RV hookup

ELEVATION: 5,478 feet

RESTRICTIONS: *Pets:* On leash at all times, strictly enforced
Fires: No ground fires whatsoever; charcoal or wood fires in pedestal grills unless high winds exist or Stage II fire restrictions are in effect; propane grills are permitted during Stage II fire restrictions
Alcohol: No alcohol permitted whatsoever
Quiet Hours: 10 p.m.–8 a.m.
Stay Limit: 14 days
Other: Gates are locked from 10 p.m.–6 a.m. every night; gate combination code will be issued at check in

MAP

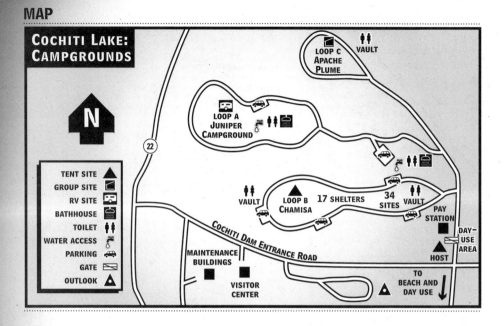

COCHITI LAKE: CAMPGROUNDS

LOOP C APACHE PLUME — VAULT

LOOP A JUNIPER CAMPGROUND

22

TENT SITE
GROUP SITE
RV SITE
BATHHOUSE
TOILET
WATER ACCESS
PARKING
GATE
OUTLOOK

VAULT

LOOP B CHAMISA — 17 SHELTERS — 34 SITES — VAULT

PAY STATION

DAY-USE AREA

HOST

MAINTENANCE BUILDINGS

COCHITI DAM ENTRANCE ROAD

VISITOR CENTER

TO BEACH AND DAY USE

GPS COORDINATES

MAIN CAMPGROUND
UTM Zone (WGS84) 13S
Easting 38003.10
Northing 3945102.18
Latitude N 35° 38" 32.84"
Longtitude W 106° 19' 31.48"

TETILLA PEAK CAMPGROUND
UTM Zone (WGS84) 13S
Easting 381703.19
Northing 3945430.80
Latitude N 35° 38" 44.23"
Longtitude W 106° 18' 24.19"

GETTING THERE

MAIN CAMPGROUND:
From Interstate 25, take Exit 264, drive northwest on NM 22 for 12 miles to Cochiti Dam entrance.

TETILLA PEAK:
From I-25, take Exit 264, drive northwest on NM 22 for 8 miles; follow NM 16 for 10 miles to Tetilla Peak entrance.

MAP

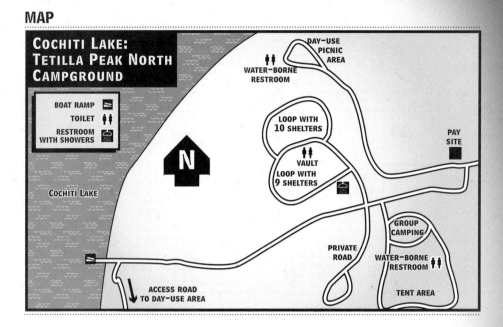

COCHITI LAKE:
TETILLA PEAK NORTH
CAMPGROUND

BOAT RAMP
TOILET
RESTROOM
WITH SHOWERS

DAY-USE
PICNIC
AREA

WATER-BORNE
RESTROOM

COCHITI LAKE

N

LOOP WITH
10 SHELTERS

VAULT
LOOP WITH
9 SHELTERS

PAY
SITE

GROUP
CAMPING

PRIVATE
ROAD

WATER-BORNE
RESTROOM

TENT AREA

ACCESS ROAD
TO DAY-USE AREA

five water spigots distributed at equal distances throughout the campground. The campground has two vault toilets, and a waterborne restroom with a shower.

Cochiti Lake has a beautiful, new sand swimming beach with covered sun shelters, but no lifeguard is present. Pets are not allowed at the beach. I have paddled my raft all over this lake, and it is a fun, clean lake. The lake is a no-wake lake, strictly enforced. Mandatory U.S. Coast Guard–approved life vests are required on the lake everywhere except the swimming beach.

Within a 6-mile drive is the Kasha-Katuwe Tent Rocks National Monument, managed by the Bureau of Land Management. This is a must-see for the Cochiti camper. Take NM 22 to the base of the dam, turn west onto Cochiti Reservation Road 84, and follow the sign to Forest Road 266 to the small roadway office. Fees are $5 per day. The temt rocks area is 4 miles further, up Forest Road 266. There are only 3 miles of hiking trails here, and hiking is easy to moderate with a few steep areas. Be sure to hike the canyon trail, as the canyon is very narrow and incredible for photographers and artists.

While on Native American tribal land, be respectful and obey all laws.

CENTRAL NEW MEXICO
MANZANO AREA

27 CAPILLA PEAK CAMPGROUND

I **F YOU WANT A MOUNTAINTOP** camping experience, Capilla Peak is for you. You will not find a single RV up here; the road is too rough, and it is slow going in several places. The hairpin turns and the sheer cliff drop-offs along the road are not for the faint of heart, nor for those unaccustomed to heights. This road is a four-wheel-drive road, but my two-wheel-drive truck has made it a hundred times in good weather only. There are no guardrails. If it rains the road can wash out and you can get stuck in dozens of places.

And a blessing it is when you arrive. You are sitting on top of a glorious mountain, and the fresh pine air fills your lungs. You begin by staring awestruck to the east over the dramatic green Estancia Valley. You then hike to the entrance road, look to the west, and are dumbfounded by the view of the arid desert west of the town of Belen, with Mount Taylor in the distance to the west. You can see the topography of the land perfectly. On a clear day you can see clear beyond Socorro to the south.

This mountaintop can get windy. Even if it's calm in the town of Manzano where you turned off the highway, it can be an entirely different story here, so hammer those tent stakes down tight.

There are a total of eight campsites. All campsites are spacious, and privacy is good because you have large areas to pitch your tent away from other campers. In the center of the loop is a vault toilet and a large gazebo, which comes in handy when it rains.

The east loop of the campground has three Adirondack shelters. The north loop has several level campsites in a grassy meadow shaded by trees. The east side of the loop has several shady tent areas, but they aren't quite as level.

Each of the campsites come with a bear-proof food

> *The fresh pine air fills your lungs and refreshes your spirit.*

RATINGS

Beauty: ✪ ✪ ✪ ✪ ✪
Privacy: ✪ ✪ ✪ ✪ ✪
Spaciousness: ✪ ✪ ✪ ✪ ✪
Quiet: ✪ ✪ ✪ ✪ ✪
Security: ✪ ✪ ✪
Cleanliness: ✪ ✪ ✪ ✪ ✪

box, a fire pit, and a picnic table. The trash receptacles are bear proof. There are some concrete patio structures in the north and east tent areas, which make a really nice dining area. If the wind kicks up, dowse your fire. There is no water here; you have to haul in your own. Make sure you bring enough to drown your fire.

The fire tower is a short walk from the campground, and visitors are encouraged to climb up and enjoy the full 360-degree view. There is also a hiking trail nearby, but it's for foot and equestrian traffic only; no mountain bikes are allowed. ATV and motorcycle trail riders cannot ride here. There are some trails that are legal to ride near New Canyon Campground further down the mountain.

As far as security is concerned, you will see occasional patrols by the Forest Service, but I have never seen a Torrance County Sheriff here. There are fewer visitors here, which makes it safer. There is no campground host.

Come well supplied because the 12-mile drive takes almost 45 minutes each way. If you need firewood, Manzano has a wood yard; ask for alligator juniper because it burns the best of any wood they sell. The Manzano Tiendita grocery store carries a good supply of what you might need. Their prices are reasonable, and they are delightful folks.

KEY INFORMATION

ADDRESS: Mountainair Ranger District
P.O. Box 69
Mountainair, NM 87036
(505) 847-2990
Cibola National Forest Office (Albuquerque)
2113 Osuna Rd NE
Albuquerque, NM 87113
(505) 346-3900; www.fs.fed.us/r3/cibola

OPERATED BY: Mountainair Ranger District
Cibola National Forest
U.S. Department of Agriculture

OPEN: April 1–November 1, weather permitting

SITES: 8 individual sites; all sites are first come, first served

EACH SITE HAS: Parking space, picnic table, and fire ring; 3 campsites have Adirondack shelters

REGISTRATION: Self-service registration, immediately upon selecting campsite

FEE: $7 per night single unit

ELEVATION: 9,283 feet

RESTRICTIONS: *Pets:* on leash, 6-foot maximum; take precautionary measures for predators
Fires: Wood fires permitted only in provided fire rings. Charcoal grills are permitted
Quiet times: 10 p.m.–8 a.m.
Alcohol: Within campsite only
Stay Limit: 14 days
Other: Bring your own firewood, because the mountaintop has been picked clean. It needs to be mentioned again that if the wind kicks up, dowse the fire.

MAP

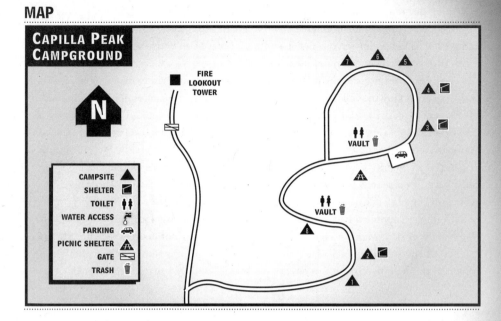

CAPILLA PEAK CAMPGROUND

FIRE LOOKOUT TOWER

N

CAMPSITE
SHELTER
TOILET
WATER ACCESS
PARKING
PICNIC SHELTER
GATE
TRASH

VAULT

VAULT

UTM Zone 13S

Easting 0371528.1

Northing 3480683.0

Latitude 41." 57.6

Longtitude 106° 24' 9.8"

GETTING THERE

From NM 55, turn west at the Capilla Peak sign onto Forest Service 245. There will be two forks; take the left fork both times. Follow the road up the mountain and drive slowly. There are a few areas where the road gets narrow and two vehicles cannot pass one another. The campground is up past the cell towers. At the top of the mountain, turn right into the campground. It is 11.4 miles from the town of Manzano to the campground.

> *You can view oaks turning brilliant reds, oranges, and yellows with groves of aspen nearby.*

NEW **CANYON CAMPGROUND** is a quaint little campground that most people drive past on the way to Capilla Peak. Being overlooked might possibly be the main appeal to this pretty campground. New Canyon is set alongside scenic Forest Service 245. From the tiny hamlet of Manzano, it's a 5-mile drive to the camp. The road is rough in several areas; although four-wheel drive is recommended, high clearance vehicles can make it if the road is not muddy. The road gets dusty during dry weather and nearly impassable after heavy rains.

October is an ideal time to camp here, with the oaks turning brilliant reds, oranges, and yellows. Several small groves of aspen can be seen nearby. Spring and summer are lovely times to camp here as well, with many species of wildflowers abounding throughout the forest. During the rainy season, a small creek intermittently flows across the road. Wild turkeys are frequently seen in this area, and mule deer, foxes, black bear, mountain lion, coyote, and elk inhabit the area.

Eight campsites are set under a tall canopy of ponderosa pine, spruce, and douglas fir, with gambel oak trees interspersed. Two other campsites are set alongside the road just to the east of the main camp. Each campsite has a picnic table and fire ring. A vault toilet is provided, as are varmint-proof trash receptacles. There is no water, so bring enough to dowse your fire. There is little to no security, but Mountainair District Rangers patrol this road occasionally. Road traffic is never too heavy during the day, and almost non-existent at night. Various species of owls inhabit the area, and perform nightly, along with an active pack of coyote.

Numerous trailheads nearby provide excellent hiking, ranging from easy to difficult. New Canyon Trailhead 101 begins at the campground; the 2-mile

RATINGS

Beauty: ☆ ☆ ☆ ☆
Privacy: ☆ ☆ ☆ ☆
Spaciousness: ☆ ☆ ☆
Quiet: ☆ ☆ ☆ ☆
Security: ☆
Cleanliness: ☆ ☆ ☆

moderate hike leads to Crest Trail 170. Crest Trail 170 is the backbone trail of the Manzano Mountain Wilderness. From the intersection of trails 101 and 170, a more strenuous hike north to Capilla Peak takes you 2.6 miles, providing the most breathtaking panoramas of the Manzano Mountains. Capilla Peak can be reached 4 miles north of the campground up FS 245. The road is rough, narrow, and there are no guardrails. After arriving at the 9,200-foot summit, you will discover the drive is worth every bump.

The nearest grocery store, Manzano Tiendita, is right along NM 337 in Manzano. This pleasant little store sells basic staples and a few items for campers. Five miles south of Manzano, and 1 mile west of the tiny town of Punta de Agua, is Quarai Pueblo Mission. Quarai is one of three ruins of the Salinas Pueblo Missions National Monument, operated by the National Park Service. The Pueblo Mission ruins are well preserved, dating back to the 1580s. Admission is free, and remember your camera.

KEY INFORMATION

ADDRESS: Cibola National Forest Mountainair Ranger District P.O. Box 69 40 Ranger Station Road Mountainair, NM 87036-0069 (505)346-3900 www.fs.fed.us/r3/ cibola/recreation/ rec-mtair.shtml

OPERATED BY: Cibola National Forest Mountainair Ranger District

OPEN: Official season, April 1–November 31, weather permitting

SITES: 10 individual sites; all sites are first come, first served

EACH SITE HAS: Parking space, picnic table, and fire ring

FEE: No fees

ELEVATION: 7,797 feet

RESTRICTIONS: *Pets:* Take precautionary measures for predators
Fires: Wood fires permitted only in provided fire rings; charcoal grills are permitted
Alcohol: Within campsite only
Stay Limit: 14 days

MAP

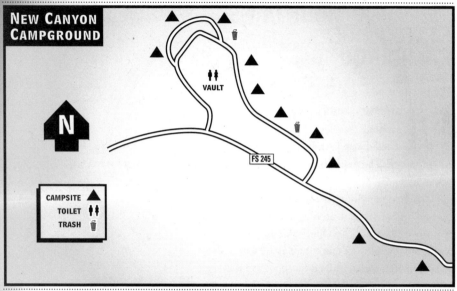

New Canyon Campground

VAULT

N

CAMPSITE ▲
TOILET ♦♦
TRASH 📧

FS 245

GETTING THERE

From Manzano turn at sign
west onto FS 245 and drive
5 miles to the campground.
Campground is on the right
side of the road.

GPS COORDINATES

UTM Zone (WGS84) 13S
Easting 0370764
Northing 3837499
Latitude 34° 40' 16.7"
Longtitude 106° 24' 38.1"

29
MANZANO MOUNTAINS STATE PARK CAMPGROUND

MANZANO **M**OUNTAINS **IS ONE** of the loveliest of all the New Mexico state parks and is located just 51 miles from the city limits of Albuquerque. The entire drive south on NM 337 is beautiful.

Drought conditions being extreme, Manzano Mountains Sate Park nearly burned in a wild fire. On Noember 19, 2007, The Ojo Peak Fire started south of Red Canyon, burning more than 7,500 acres. The cause remains undetermined but points to a human cause. About 150 firefighters were called out to fight the blaze. On the night of Thanksgiving, Mother Nature sent several inches of snow into the area, and the fire stopped within 200 yards of the park.

Manzano is a must for tent campers and holds a secret. When you first pull into the campground, you see the park filled with RVs and wonder, "What the heck am I doing here?" Well, take heart; you are going tent camping. Follow the loop and find the gate to the right. If it's locked, the campground manager will be happy to unlock it for you. The gate stays locked unless overflow spaces are required, or if you request camping away from the RVs.

There is a beautiful gazebo set up for group camping, and you'll appreciate it if a thunderstorm hits. The campsites are dirt, but there are grassy areas set back for your tent. The area has several trash receptacles, a fire ring, and a table at each site. This is a quiet park; the RVs have electricity, and generators are not allowed.

This state park was established in 1978 and encompasses 160 acres. Several easy nature trails meander through the park. The water system is pressurized, and the state park regularly checks and treats the water. There is a trace of chlorine, so filtering is wise. There are 16 developed campsites in the RV loop and 31 primitive campsites in the overflow and

> *One of the loveliest of all New Mexico State Parks*

RATINGS

Beauty: ✩ ✩ ✩ ✩ ✩
Privacy: ✩ ✩ ✩ ✩
Spaciousness: ✩ ✩ ✩ ✩
Quiet: ✩ ✩ ✩ ✩ ✩
Security: ✩ ✩ ✩ ✩ ✩
Cleanliness: ✩ ✩ ✩ ✩ ✩

ADDRESS: Manzano Mountains
State Park
HC-66, Box 202
Mountainair, NM
87036
(505) 344-7240
www.emnrd.state
.nm.us/PRD

OPERATED BY: New Mexico State
Parks, New Mexico
Energy
Minerals and
Natural Resources
Department

OPEN: April 1–November 1

EACH SITE HAS: Parking space, picnic table, and fire
ring; developed sites
have water, sewer; 8
sites have electricity

REGISTRATION: Self-service
registration,
immediately upon
selecting campsite

FEE: $10 per night devel-
oped or primitive,
$4 electricity fee,
$4 sewer fee; water
hookup is free; for
group camping
contact park for
reservations and fee

ELEVATION: 8,376 feet

RESTRICTIONS: *Pets:* On leash, 6-foot
maximum
Fires: Wood fires
permitted only in
provided fire rings;
charcoal grills are
permitted
Alcohol: Within
campsite only
Quiet Hours: 10 p.m.–
8 a.m.
Stay Limit: 14 days
Other: gate hours,
7:30 a.m.–sunset

group area. The restrooms are sparkling clean with flush toilets and sinks but no showers. With a new staff residence opening in spring of 2008, this park is tenta-tiviley slated to open year round.

This camp is very secure. The campground man-ager lives on-site and regular patrols are made by New Mexico Parks Department law enforcement officers and the Torrance County Sheriff's Department.

The park office is open on weekends and loans reading material on the plants and animals endemic to the area. You can also obtain a list of bird species that are native to the park. Stellar's jays and Albert's squir-rels are quite entertaining and easy to photograph at the feeders in front of the park office. Bring your hum-mingbird feeder; you will be happy you did.

The Manzano Mountains are a great place to be if you love birds. It is a main migratory flyway and many raptors follow the waterfowl back and forth. Nearby Capilla Peak has a raptor viewing area that is worth a visit.

The forest here is a mixture of ponderosa, pinon, gambel oak, emory oak, and alligator juniper. The alli-gator juniper is named for the checkered pattern on the bark of older trees, which resembles an alligator's hide. The name *Manzano* means "apple tree" in Span-ish, but there are no apple trees here. However, if you hike back into the forest, there are plenty of pinon nuts you can gather for a healthy camp snack.

The apple trees in the Manzano Mountains were planted by Spanish missionaries throughout this area in the 1800s. These remaining trees may be the oldest living apple trees in the United States.

There is no firewood at this campground; the for-est has been picked clean. There is a wood yard on the main highway, at the state park turnoff road. Buy some alligator juniper; it is great burning firewood, and the wood itself has a beautiful scent to it.

Be prepared to cold camp during the dry seasons. The Manzano Mountains get far less precipitation (14.2 inches per year) than the mountains in Northern New Mexico. When fire restrictions go into effect in the adjacent Cibola National Forest, this state park takes the same action. Every year Stage II fire restrictions

MAP

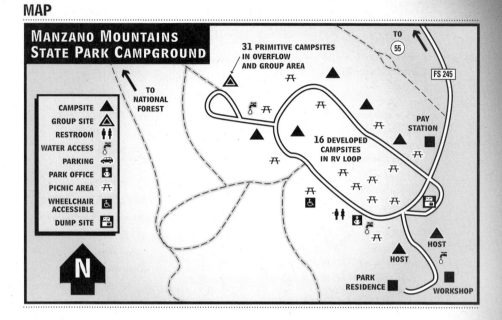

MANZANO MOUNTAINS STATE PARK CAMPGROUND

31 PRIMITIVE CAMPSITES IN OVERFLOW AND GROUP AREA

TO 55

FS 245

TO NATIONAL FOREST

CAMPSITE
GROUP SITE
RESTROOM
WATER ACCESS
PARKING
PARK OFFICE
PICNIC AREA
WHEELCHAIR ACCESSIBLE
DUMP SITE

PAY STATION

16 DEVELOPED CAMPSITES IN RV LOOP

HOST

HOST

PARK RESIDENCE

WORKSHOP

N

are a reality here, but don't let that discourage you from camping here.

The Manzano Mountains are substantially warmer than the mountains to the north. Because of this, all of the campgrounds open in April. I was delighted to wake up to a beautiful six-inch snowfall here in late April of 2006. It melted fast, and the mercury rose to 60°F by noon.

The Manzano Tiendita store on Highway 55 carries adequate groceries, but not many camping supplies; the prices are reasonable.

Five miles south of Manzano is a town named Punte de Agua. The Quarai Ruins, part of the Salinas Pueblo Missions National Monument, are just 1 mile west of Punte de Agua. The Tiwa Pueblo here was already in existence in 1529 when Spanish explorer Juan de Onate discovered it in 1598. The mission was established in 1629. Other nearby attractions are a breathtaking drive to the top of Capilla Peak and the Tajique/Torreon horseshoe drive down Forest Service 55 near Tajique.

GETTING THERE

From NM 337 in Manzano, turn right at the Manzano Mountains State Park sign, following FS 245 for 3 miles. When the asphalt road turns to the right, follow the gravel road straight, and Manzano is just ahead at the top of the hill.

GPS COORDINATES

UTM Zone (WGS84) 13S
Easting 0375201.1
Northing 3829931.0
Latitude N34° 36' 13.07"
Longtitude W106° 21' 39.78"

> *Semi-remote and very beautiful*

RED CANYON CAMPGROUND is situated in a tall forest of ponderosa pine, with scattered fir, spruce, and aspen. I have been there dozens of times and have never seen this campground full. The real attraction is that it's under-used. This campground is semi-remote and is very beautiful. The dirt road to Red Canyon has a few bumpy spots, and thus not recommended for cars but is well maintained.

Due to extreme drought conditions, Red Canyon nearly became a victim of a wild fire. On November 19, 2007, The Ojo Peak Fire started south of Red Canyon, burning more than 7,500 acres. The cause remains undetermined but points to a human cause. About 150 firefighters were called out to fight the blaze. On the night of Thanksgiving, Mother Nature sent several inches of snow into the Manzano Mountains, and the fire stopped right outside of the campground. Fire damage is apparent all around the campground, and several homes were destroyed in this area.

The campground is divided into two separate camps. Driving to the right up hill, you find the equestrian camp with parking for trailers and corrals for horses. The lower camp, 50 yards further to the south, is for tent campers and RVs. Several easy-to-moderate hiking trails are here, and the trail information is posted right at the trailhead in the campground.

There is no water available at the camp, but you can fill up at Manzano Mountains State Park 3 miles away. Filter the water, as it is treated with chlorine. There are 18 campsites at the equestrian camp and 20 sites at the lower camp. There is usually an RV or two here, but it is quiet overall. This is a good campground to choose if you wish for serenity and peace. Each campsite is equipped with a fire ring and picnic table. The pit toilets are in good condition and clean. There is no campground host here, and there may be a patrol

RATINGS

Beauty: ☆ ☆ ☆ ☆ ☆
Privacy: ☆ ☆ ☆ ☆ ☆
Spaciousness: ☆ ☆ ☆ ☆
Quiet: ☆ ☆ ☆ ☆ ☆
Security: ☆
Cleanliness: ☆ ☆ ☆ ☆ ☆

by the U.S. Forest Service or the Torrance County Sheriff's Department, but don't count on much security.

This campground is protected by the mountain on two sides and a tall canopy of ponderosa pines. When it gets windy, you are well protected. All campsites provide liberal shade. When it rains, a mud bog forms in the center of the campground due to poor drainage. A better choice is selecting a campsite on the outside of the loops where the runoff is better.

Cibola National Forest began timber thinning at this camp in 2006. There is plenty of firewood. As in all national forests, it is mandatory to carry a shovel and axe. Be careful with your campfire, because the only water available is what you carry.

Due to this remote location, black bear, mountain lion, bobcat, and coyote are common here, as are raccoons. There are no bear-proof food boxes here, so keep your food in the vehicle. The trash receptacles are bear proof. Read and comply with the bear-alert postings and you will be safe.

There is occasionally stagnant water in the streambed, so mosquitoes might be an occasional problem. Deer and elk droppings are also found frequently here, so beware of deer ticks.

You'll find several nearby attractions while camping here. Five miles south of Manzano is a town named Punte de Agua. There is a small park here with a gazebo and a windmill pressurizing the well. The quality of the water is unknown.

KEY INFORMATION

ADDRESS:	Cibola National Forest, Albuquerque Office
	2113 Osuna Road, NE, Suite A
	Albuquerque, NM 87113
	Albuquerque office phone: (505) 346-3900
	Mountainair Ranger District Office
	P.O. Box 69
	Mountainair, NM 87036
	Mountainair office phone: (505) 847-2990; www.fs.fed.us/r3/cibola
OPERATED BY:	Mountainair Ranger District, Cibola National Forest
OPEN:	Official season, Memorial Day–Labor Day
SITES:	38 individual sites; all sites are on a first-come, first-serve basis
EACH SITE HAS:	Parking space, picnic table, and fire ring
REGISTRATION:	Self-service registration, immediately upon selecting campsite
FEE:	$7 per night single unit
ELEVATION:	8,376 feet
RESTRICTIONS:	*Pets:* On leash, 6-foot maximum; take precautionary measures for predators
	Fires: Wood fires permitted only in provided fire rings; charcoal grills are permitted
	Alcohol: Within campsite only
	Quiet times: 10 p.m.–8 a.m.
	Stay Limit: 14 days

MAP

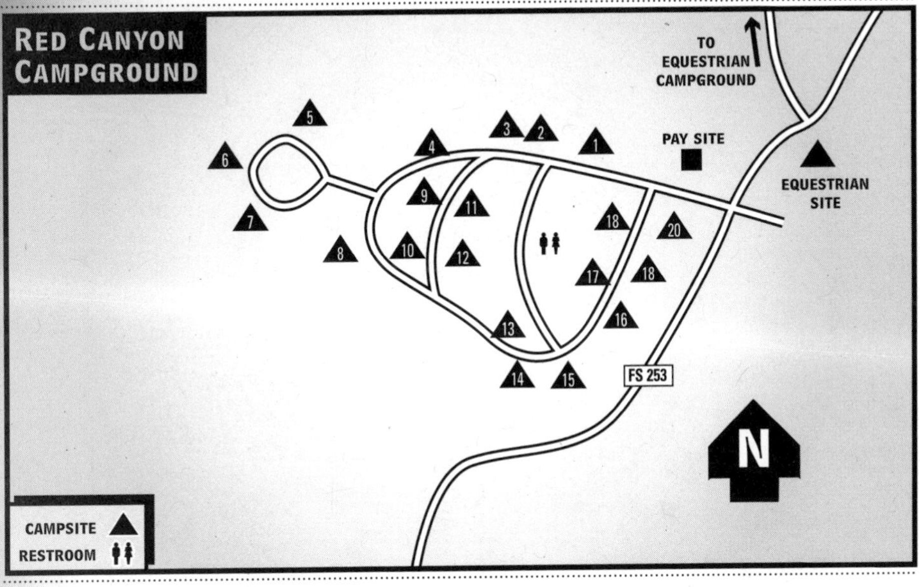
RED CANYON CAMPGROUND
TO EQUESTRIAN CAMPGROUND
PAY SITE
EQUESTRIAN SITE
FS 253
N
CAMPSITE
RESTROOM

GETTING THERE

From the town of Manzano, follow the road signs leading to Manzano Mountains State Park. This is Forest Service 253. Stay on FS 253 for 3 miles until you arrive at the Manzano Mountains State Park entrance sign. At this three-way intersection, the road turns 90 degrees. Turn right and stay on this road. From the three-way intersection, it is another 3 miles to the entrances.

The road veers to the right and up the hill to the equestrian camp. The main campground entrance is only 50 yards ahead.

Don't miss the Quarai Ruins, part of the Salinas Pueblo Missions National Monument. The ruins are 12 miles from the campground. The Tiwa Pueblo here was already in existence in 1529 when Spanish explorer Juan de Onate discovered it in 1598. The mission was established in 1629. Two other attractions nearby are a breathtaking 12-mile drive to the top of Capilla Peak up FS 245 and the Tajique/Torreon horseshoe drive on FS 55.

The Manzano Tiendita convenience store carries adequate groceries, but few camping supplies. The prices are reasonable, and the owners are friendly.

GPS COORDINATES

UTM Zone (WGS84) 13S
Easting 371355.0
Northing 383135.5
Latitude 34° 36' 58"
Longtitude 106° 24' 12"

CENTRAL NEW MEXICO
TAJIQUE AREA

31
FOURTH OF JULY CAMPGROUND

> *Tent camper's paradise . . . with lots of hiking trails*

IF THERE EVER WAS A PARADISE for tent campers, Fourth of July Campground has to be the one. The sign at the entrance, "RV Camping at Red Canyon Campground," is the first thing that directs the big rigs to another location; small parking spots is the other. Most parking places are just large enough for a car. Pop-up campers are welcome in this campground, but it would be a tight squeeze getting a pop-up camper and a tow vehicle into one space. The campground host site is set up at the entrance of the campground and has electricity. His is the only hard-sided RV allowed in the camp.

Camping spots are well-shaded in a forest of ponderosa pine, spruce, alligator juniper, pinon, big-toothed maple, aspen, and gambel oak trees. This campground is well designed for tents, although some campsites are spaced closely together. Most areas provide enough spacing to afford privacy. There is plenty of room to set your tent back and away from others.

I motorcycle camped here in 2006, walked through on a scouting visit in March of 2007, and I noticed on each trip that Forest Service 55 is well maintained, because there are areas adjacent to the forest that are privately owned. FS 55 is an absolutely magnificent drive, and the entire road is 17 miles in length.

This is a magnificent campground. The cinder-block vault toilets are modern, with solar-powered lighting. Both loops are fairly long, the round-trip for a bicycle is three-quarters of a mile. It is a great campground for kids; they will have lots of room to play.

Three trailheads are located within the campground: Albuquerque, Fourth of July, and Mosca. These trails are rated as moderate, and range from 0.8 of a mile to 3.5 miles in length. There is a parking lot specifically for hikers at the campground entrance. Trail maps are available at the pay station. Day-use

RATINGS

Beauty: ✰ ✰ ✰ ✰ ✰
Privacy: ✰ ✰ ✰
Spaciousness: ✰ ✰ ✰
Quiet: ✰ ✰ ✰
Security: ✰ ✰ ✰ ✰ ✰
Cleanliness: ✰ ✰ ✰ ✰ ✰

and hiking fees are $5 per day. Incidentally, this is a great place to launch backpacking trips. No mountain bikes or off-road vehicles are allowed on the trails.

The two camping loops are named Gallo and Masca. Both loops have two vault toilet buildings each, and bear-proof trash cans. Gallo has smaller campsites, so check Masca first if you want a roomier area. Gallo curves off to the left with 16 single sites. Masca Loop has five single sites, one double site with two tables and two fire rings, and and one triple site with three tables and three fire rings. All single sites have a fire ring, table, and a parking spot. This campground is very secure; a campground host is assigned here from Memorial Day through Labor day. Frequent patrols are made by the Forest Service and Torrance County Sheriff's Department.

The campground opens April 1 through November 1. Camping here before Memorial Day and after Labor Day is awesome. It gets cool at night, sometimes reaching the low 40s. Black bear, mountain lion, bobcat, and coyote are common, so obey the posted alerts. Occasional rattlesnakes have been spotted, so watch your kids and pets closely.

There is no firewood available. There is no water here either; you have to haul in your own, so make sure you bring enough water to dowse your fire. Firewood and a water tap are available at Ray's General Store, 7 miles away in the sleepy little town of Tajique. The store is well stocked with groceries and liquor and sells gasoline. The store carries portable propane bottles and picnic supplies but no camping gear. The family that runs the store is nice, and the prices are reasonable.

KEY INFORMATION

ADDRESS: Mountainair Ranger District P.O. Box 69 Mountainair, NM 87036 (505) 847-2990 or (505) 346-3900 www.fs.fed.us/r3/cibola

OPERATED BY: Mountainair Ranger District, Cibola National Forest, U.S. Department of Agriculture

OPEN: April 1– November 1

SITES: 23 individual sites; all sites are first come, first served

EACH SITE: Parking space, picnic table, and fire ring; there is no water in this campground

REGISTRATION: Self-service registration, immediately upon selecting campsite

FEE: $7 per night single site; $14 per night double site; $21 per night triple site

ELEVATION: 7,493 feet

RESTRICTIONS: *Pets:* On leash, 6-foot maximum; take precautionary measures for predators
Fires: Wood fires permitted only in provided fire rings; charcoal grills are permitted
Alcohol: Within campsite only
Quiet times: 10 p.m.– 8 a.m.
Stay limit: 14 days

MAP

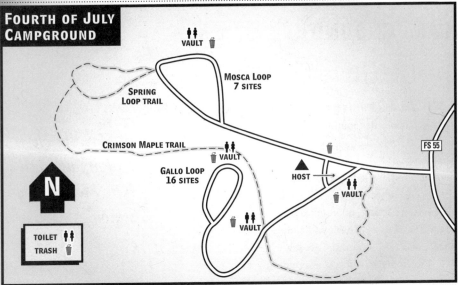

FOURTH OF JULY CAMPGROUND

VAULT

MOSCA LOOP
7 SITES

SPRING
LOOP TRAIL

CRIMSON MAPLE TRAIL

VAULT

GALLO LOOP
16 SITES

HOST

VAULT

N

VAULT

VAULT

TOILET
TRASH

FS 55

GETTING THERE

From NM 337 at the town of Tajique, turn at the campground sign, and follow FS 55 7 miles to the campground.

GPS COORDINATES

UTM Zone 13S
Easting 0373893.4
Northing 3850597.9
Latitude 34° 47' 23.26"
Longtitude 106° 22' 42.22"

32
TAJIQUE
CAMPGROUND

A SMALL, PRETTY CAMPGROUND awaits you just a few miles southwest of the tiny hamlet of Tajique. Tajique (pronounced: tuh-hee-kee) Campground has only five sites but is a comfortable campground nestled right off Forest Service 55. During the spring snowmelt, tiny Tajique Creek flows freely. There is no fishing, but it gives the campground a magical ambience. In May, the creek will dry up until the New Mexico monsoon season.

Enveloped in a forest of ponderosa pine, red cedar, pinon, alligator juniper, and gambel oak, the entire campground is shady. Outside of traffic passing on FS 55, the campground remains relatively quiet. This is one of those campgrounds for tents, not RVs, and because of the parking configuration, the loop is too small for RV parking.

There are five campsites, three along the loop and two more tucked back in the woods. Four of the five campsites have picnic tables and fire grates. The campsite to the right as you turn in is not very appealing (it will catch a fair amount of dust from the road), but the other four sites sit back from the road. This is a popular campground, and there are many areas to set your tent up by the grassy streambed.

There is a beautiful site across the stream, an easy 50-foot walk from the end of the loop. It sits apart from the other campsites and could be considered a "honeymoon suite," not visible from the campground loop. The other remote campsite is a 100-foot walk east of the vault toilet. This site has a rock fire ring but no picnic table.

This campground is a delight to camp in if everyone keeps it clean. There is no water, so bring an adequate supply of water to dowse your campfire. There are a few short trails around the campground. All of the campsites are a decent size, and there is adequate

> *In May, the creek will dry up until the New Mexico monsoon season.*

RATINGS

Beauty: ☆ ☆ ☆ ☆
Privacy: ☆ ☆ ☆ ☆
Spaciousness: ☆ ☆ ☆ ☆ ☆
Quiet: ☆ ☆ ☆
Security: ☆ ☆ ☆
Cleanliness: ☆ ☆ ☆ ☆ ☆

ADDRESS: Mountainair Ranger District
P.O. Box 69
Mountainair, NM 87036
(505) 847-2990
www.fs.fed.us/r3/cibola

OPERATED BY: Mountainair Ranger District
Cibola National Forest
U.S. Department of Agriculture

OPEN: Year-round

SITES: 5 individual sites; all sites are first come, first served

EACH SITE: Fire ring, 4 sites have tables. Loop has adequate parking for no more than 5 vehicles

FEE: None

ELEVATION: 6,974 feet

RESTRICTIONS: *Pets:* On leash, 6-foot maximum; take precautionary measures for predators
Fires: Wood fires permitted only in provided fire rings; charcoal grills are permitted
Alcohol: No restrictions
Stay Limit: 14 days

space for privacy. Kids enjoy this campground because there is plenty of room to play. The loop is too small for bicycle riding, but kids can bike the trails.

Because of the stream, beware of black bears, mountain lion, bobcat, raccoon, and coyote. Needless to say, be sure to lock up all food items at night. Diamondback and prairie rattlesnakes inhabit the forests, so rein in the pets.

There are nearby hiking trails but none in walking distance. The road outside the park gets quite dusty in the summer, and vehicles are known to speed along FS 55 at quite a clip, so beware.

The vault toilet is in good condition; there is no vandalism, and the facility is clean. There is no host and no fee, but there are bear-proof trash receptacles. Forest Service officers patrol this area with some regularity, as does the Torrance County Sheriff's Department.

The place has been picked clean of firewood. In the town of Tajique, Ray's General Store sells pinon and cedar firewood. It is well stocked for groceries and liquor. It sells gasoline and picnic supplies but no camping gear. The prices are reasonable.

MAP

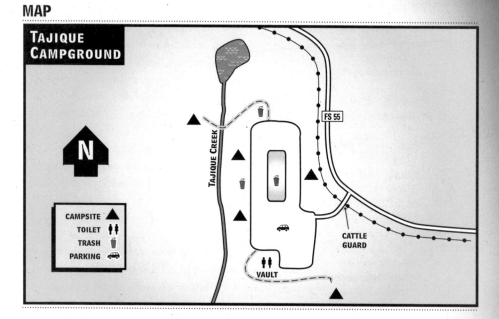

TAJIQUE CAMPGROUND

N

TAJIQUE CREEK

FS 55

CATTLE GUARD

VAULT

CAMPSITE
TOILET
TRASH
PARKING

GETTING THERE

From NM 337 at Tajique, turn west onto FS 55 at the Fourth of July Campground sign. Drive 3 miles and turn left into the campground.

GPS COORDINATES

UTM Zone 13S
Easting 0378542
Northing 3847609
Latitude 34° 45' 48"
Longtitude 106° 19' 38"

SOUTH CENTRAL
STATE PARKS

33
CABALLO LAKE
STATE PARK

WHEN PEOPLE THINK of lake camping in New Mexico, Elephant Butte Lake is the first place mentioned. But Elephant Butte is crowded, overdeveloped, and "party central." A quieter choice is lovely Caballo Lake State Park, just 16 miles south of Elephant Butte. Caballo is New Mexico's third largest state park and much more serene. Caballo campgrounds fill rapidly on the holidays, but tent campers can always find space.

Caballo Lake was formed by an earth-filled dam that is 96 feet high and 4,558 feet long. Although Caballo Lake is shallow with an average depth of 25 feet, the water surface area covers 11,500 acres and measures 18 miles long when at capacity. Depending on drought conditions, spillway gates are closed to preserve the precious water. During the summer, the floodgates open to provide the fertile Mesilla (pronounced muh-see-uh) Valley, a few miles to the south, much needed irrigation. This is where the delicious New Mexico green and red chile is grown, along with many other crops. The Mesilla Valley is lush and green, a lovely oasis in the south-central New Mexico desert.

The Caballo Lake staff manages the crowds here well. The Sierra County Sheriff's Department and the New Mexico State Police patrol the campgrounds regularly. The U.S. Coast Guard Auxiliary has staff stationed here, and state park officers patrol the lake constantly. Pick up a boater's safety brochure because New Mexico boating laws have changed recently and are strictly enforced. This beautiful desert lake is a boater's paradise; popular for fishing, water skiing, windsurfing, canoeing, kayaking, and inflatables.

For tent campers, the best sites are found at Riverside Campground, on the south end of the dam. This is tent camping at its finest. From the entrance point of this campground to the loop at the far end is exactly

> *Riverside campsites are shady with Russian olive, cottonwood, and salt cedar trees.*

RATINGS

Beauty: ✩ ✩ ✩ ✩
Privacy: ✩ ✩ ✩
Spaciousness: ✩ ✩ ✩
Quiet: ✩ ✩ ✩ ✩
Security: ✩ ✩ ✩ ✩ ✩
Cleanliness: ✩ ✩ ✩ ✩ ✩

ADDRESS: Caballo Lake State
Park
P.O. Box 32
Caballo, NM 87931
(505) 743-3942
www.emnrd.state.nm
.us/PRD/caballo.
htm.Visitor center
hours 8 a.m.–6 p.m.

OPERATED BY: New Mexico State
Parks

OPEN: Year-round

SITES: 135 individual sites;
tent sites are first
come, first served;
for reservations,
visit www.nmparks
.com, or call
(877) NM4-RSVP

EACH SITE HAS: Developed sites
have parking space,
picnic table, and fire
ring

REGISTRATION: Registration at
visitor center or self-
service registration

FEE: $8 primitive site;
$10 developed site;
$4 electrical hookup;
$4 sewage hookup

ELEVATION: 4,172 feet (Riverside); 4,259 feet
(Lake Office)

RESTRICTIONS: *Pets:* On leash,
strictly enforced;
take precautionary
measures for
predators
Fires: Wood fires in
fire rings; charcoal
grills permitted
Alcohol: Zero
tolerance while
boating, permitted
at campsite only
Quiet Hours: 10 p.m.–
8 a.m.
Stay Limit: 14 days

1 mile. Almost all of the tent spots are located between the road and the Rio Grande. The riverside campsites are shady, with a mix of Russian olive, cottonwood, and salt cedar trees. The ground is level and sandy with sparse wild grasses. You can pitch your tent right under the trees. The Youth Conservation Corps worked hard to install dozens of new shelters throughout the entire campground. Primitive camping is permitted here, and many sites are available without a picnic table or fire grate, but ground fires are not permitted. There is one comfort station equipped with full flush toilets, sinks, and showers. One water spigot is located in front of the comfort station; 50 feet to the north is a modern playground.

Past the visitor center in the lakeside area are five camping areas for RV's separated from the tent areas. Two primitive camping areas are available for tent campers. Percha Flats Campground is located on the southwest corner of the lake below the dam. If the ground is dry, it makes for ideal beach camping. This is a large area for dispersed camping, but there are no picnic tables, fire rings, or toilets; and there is no shade, RVs are across the road and have a full hookup and water at each site, and generator use is not permitted.

North of the boat dock, Upper Flats Beach Campground provides dispersed primitive camping with a few picnic tables and fire grates but little shade. Three portable outhouses are in this area.

You'll find an incredible cactus garden at the visitor center. The wide variety of cacti bloom in April and May. More than 200 species of birds and waterfowl thrive here, including the sandhill crane. Bald eagle, and golden eagle roost here seasonally, following the waterfowl migrations. Turkey vultures are a common sight, scavenging for fish. The park is home to coyote, several squirrel species, rabbits, foxes, raccoons, mule deer, black bear, rattlesnakes, lizards, frogs, and turtles. Bobcat and mountain lion have been spotted in the Caballo Mountains, but fight shy of the park.

In summer, you can expect temperatures in the 100°F range, but it cools down to the 70s at night. Thunderstorms are rare until July, when the monsoon season is welcomed here in the Chihuahuan Desert. The sunsets are incredible; the pink and orange hori-

MAP

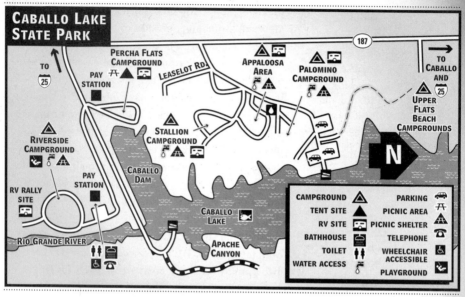

zon sets the Caballo Mountains a fiery red nearly every evening. The night skies are wide open, and it's a stargazer's paradise, so bring your telescope.

GETTING THERE

Caballo is located 16 miles south of Truth or Consequences off Interstate 25, exit 59, and follow signs. There are two entrances; the north entrance leads to the visitor center and lakeside campgrounds, and the south entrance leads to the dam road and the Riverside Campground area.

GPS COORDINATES

RIVERSIDE (GATE):

UTM Zone (WGS84) 13S
Easting 0285493
Northing 3641908
Latitude 32° 53' 39.7"
Longtitude 107° 17' 35.8"

LAKESIDE (OFFICE)

UTM Zone (WGS84) 13S
Easting 0283997
Northing 3643420
Latitude 32° 54' 27.7"
Longtitude 107° 18' 34.6"

> *A hidden gem, surrounded by several farms in the lush Mesilla Valley*

PERCHA DAM STATE PARK features a beautiful, quiet, small campground located just a scant 3 miles south of Caballo Lake State Park. It is a hidden gem, surrounded by several farms in the lush Mesilla Valley. Named for Percha Creek, which flows into the Rio Grande River, the sound of water cascading over the dam can be heard throughout the campground. This serene park provides an ideal place to kick back and relax. It's a wonderful tent camper's-park.

Swimming is not recommended here because of the swift current of the Rio Grande, but canoeing, rafting, and kayaking are excellent. All occupants in the watercraft must wear a personal flotation device—no exceptions. Fishing in the small pond is fair for bass, catfish, and occasional walleye. No swimming is permitted in the nearby irrigation canals because of possible pesticide contamination in the water. The state of New Mexico has made some significant improvements here, including a modern playground at the park's south end.

Tent camping is dispersed, and there are no marked or numbered sites. Just set the tent up where you wish and enjoy the lush grass and shade of the cottonwood, river willow, russian olive, ash, and salt cedar trees. Several sites along the Rio Grande River provide excellent shade, grass, a few picnic tables, and fire rings. Several water spigots are located throughout the park. The state performs frequent water tests, but I still highly recommend that you filter this water. Plenty of parking is available.

Many dispersed tent sites lie under tall cottonwood trees in the grass meadow between the roads. These sites are on a slight downslope. Water runoff flows into a small canal dividing the meadow area in half. This meadow is ideal for tents, but there is little to no privacy here between sites. A group shelter houses

RATINGS

Beauty: ✿ ✿ ✿ ✿
Privacy: ✿ ✿
Spaciousness: ✿ ✿ ✿ ✿
Quiet: ✿ ✿ ✿ ✿
Security: ✿ ✿ ✿ ✿ ✿
Cleanliness: ✿ ✿ ✿ ✿ ✿

a dozen picnic tables and a fireplace. It provides an excellent escape from afternoon summer rains. There is no firewood here; you must bring your own.

Security is excellent. The area is patrolled by the New Mexico State Parks, New Mexico State Police, Sierra County Sheriff's Department, and New Mexico game wardens. Have your fishing license available at all times.

The park offers an immaculate comfort station equipped with flush toilets, sinks, and showers. The RV area is well separated from the tent sites, and all have electric and water hookups. Generator use is not permitted at this campground. A campground host is on-site.

If you feel like a little exercise, check out the short half-mile hiking trail within the park. The park is known as a prime bird-watcher's paradise. Among waterfowl you will see various species of ducks, geese, heron, cranes, and swans. Occasional sightings of golden and bald eagles, a variety of hawks, and falcons are common here. The elusive peregrine falcon makes its aerie in the nearby Caballo Mountains. You may spot occasional deer, coyotes, raccoons, red foxes, rabbits, and squirrels throughout the area.

Temperatures often exceed 100°F in summer, but with shade trees, summer breezes, and low humidity, it is still pleasant. Folks drive to Caballo Lake to swim or canoe for the day to escape the heat. Nights cool off into the 70s in the summer, with gentle breezes. Occasional thunderstorms begin in July and cool things off. I love walking in the warm summer rain.

The small town of Hatch, New Mexico, is 18 miles south, off Interstate 25. It's an excellent place for supplies. The town is the main entry point of the Mesilla Valley, so the produce here is incredible. In the fall apples, peaches, and apricots are available. Also try the pistachio and almond nuts grown here and sold all year. You will be amazed at the variety of New Mexico chile products to sample, including green chile chocolate candy!

KEY INFORMATION

ADDRESS: Caballo State Park
P.O. Box 32
Caballo, NM 87931
(505) 743-3942
www.emnrd.state
.nm.us/PRD/
Percha.htm

OPERATED BY: New Mexico State Parks

OPEN: Year-round

SITES: 75; primitive sites are not numbered, but there is plenty of room; all are first come, first served

EACH SITE HAS: Parking space, picnic table, and fire ring

REGISTRATION: Self-service registration, immediately upon selecting campsite

FEE: $10 per night for a developed site with picnic table and fire ring

ELEVATION: 4,149 feet

RESTRICTIONS: *Pets:* On leash (6-foot maximum)
Fires: Wood fires permitted only in fire rings; charcoal grills permitted
Alcohol: Within campsite only
Quiet Hours: 10 p.m.–8 a.m.
Stay Limit: 14 days

MAP

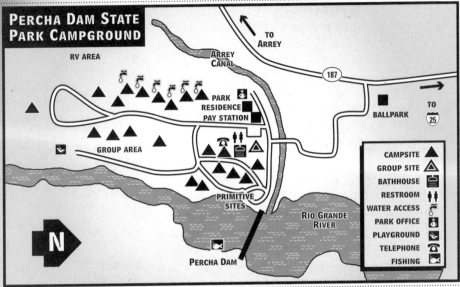

PERCHA DAM STATE PARK CAMPGROUND

RV AREA

TO ARREY

ARREY CANAL

187

PARK RESIDENCE

PAY STATION

BALLPARK

TO 25

GROUP AREA

PRIMITIVE SITES

RIO GRANDE RIVER

PERCHA DAM

N

CAMPSITE	▲
GROUP SITE	△
BATHHOUSE	
RESTROOM	
WATER ACCESS	
PARK OFFICE	
PLAYGROUND	
TELEPHONE	
FISHING	

GETTING THERE

Take I-25 to exit 59. Follow NM 159 south 2 miles, turn left at the Percha Dam sign, and follow the road 1 mile to the campground.

GPS COORDINATES

UTM Zone (WGS84) 13S
Easting 0284236
Northing 3639109
Latitude 32° 52' 08.0"
Longtitude 107° 18' 21.8"

PERCHED HIGH IN THE FOOTHILLS beneath the towering cathedral spires of the Organ Mountains, beautiful Aguirre Springs Recreation Area is a must for those who wish to experience a Chihuahuan Desert camping experience. This desert camp is the only high-country campground in the area, and is conveniently located 17 miles east of Las Cruces.

A unique Chihuahuan Desert camping experience

White Sands Missile Range and the Tularosa Valley provide majestic views to the north and east. Yucca blooms appear in April through mid-June, when native cacti and succulent plants flower at the same time. Pinon and juniper dot the rugged hillsides, adding a lovely hue of green to the gray and tan of the Organ Mountains.

Alligator juniper, gray oak, and mountain mahogany provide shade. Dwarf mesquite trees are native here. Mule deer, oryx, and pronghorn antelope are common. Visits by mountain lions have become more frequent, so beware. Pinon, cedar, alligator juniper, gray oak, and mountain mahogany provide shade. Rattlesnakes are common here, so brush up on how to avoid them. Keep your tents zipped tightly shut at all times. Several species of scorpions and centipedes are residents you will want to avoid.

In 1991 a flash flood and mudslide wiped out more than 75 percent of the campground. The Bureau of Land Management rebuilt the campground, and it remains one of the most popular campgrounds in Southeastern New Mexico.

Two hiking trails are featured in the Aguirre Springs Recreation Area; Baylor Pass Trail, 6 miles in length, takes you to the other side of the Organ Mountains. Pine Tree Trail is a 4-mile trail that takes you into ponderosa and spruce forest. Both trails offer great views of the Tularosa Basin. White Sands National Monument is 34 miles north on US 70 and

RATINGS

Beauty: ✿ ✿ ✿ ✿
Privacy: ✿ ✿ ✿
Spaciousness: ✿ ✿ ✿
Quiet: ✿ ✿ ✿ ✿
Security: ✿ ✿ ✿ ✿
Cleanliness: ✿ ✿ ✿ ✿ ✿

ADDRESS: Las Cruces District Office
1800 Marquess Street
Las Cruces, NM
88005-3370
(505) 525-4300
www.blm.gov/nm/st/
en/prog/recreation/
las_cruces/aguirre_
spring_campground
.html

OPERATED BY: Bureau of Land
Management, Las
Cruces District
Office, U.S.
Department of the
Interior

OPEN: Year-round; April–
October, entrance
gate open 8 a.m.–
8 p.m.; October–
April, 8 a.m.–6 p.m.

SITES: 57 individual sites;
all sites are first
come, first served

EACH SITE HAS: Parking space, trash
can, picnic table, fire
ring. Many sites
provide metal shel-
ters where tree
shade is lacking, and
most sites have a
pedestal grill

REGISTRATION: Self-service
registration

FEE: $3 per night

ELEVATION: 5,639 feet

RESTRICTIONS: *Pets:* On leash, 6-foot
maximum; take
precautionary
measures for
predators
Fires: Permitted in
fire rings; charcoal
grills permitted
Alcohol: At site
Quiet Hours: 10 p.m.–
8 a.m.
Stay Limit: 14 days

is a must-see. It is a playground of pure white gypsum sand and an enjoyable day trip.

The Aguirre Springs campground gets busy on weekends. Campsites serve as picnic sites for Las Cruces residents. Steel shelters provide shade in sites where trees are not present. All campsites have a picnic table, fire ring, and pedestal grills. There are three modern vault toilets in the camp. Gathering firewood is prohibited here, but firewood is sold at the campground host's residence where the water supply is located. Filtering the water is recommended.

The campground is divided into two areas, the main loop and the east loop. All campsites accommodate tents, but many of the sites in the main loop are not level. There is no grass, and the ground can be rocky in spots. The most level sites are in the east loop, and there is more privacy there away from the picnic crowds. Most sites have privacy due to trees and native desert bushes. The campground is scenic, and the early morning sunlight catches the Organ Mountains best for pictures.

The campground attracts a few RVs, but is designed for tent campers. Summers here can be quite hot, exceeding 100°F. The ideal camping season is spring, due to the blooming yucca and cacti. Fall is pleasant, but can be quite windy. Expect spring and fall daytime temperatures in the 70°F range, while nights drop into the 50s. Winter can be quite cold here, dropping as low as 20°F at night, and snow is possible anytime from November through March. Daytime temperatures in winter are 40°F to 60°F. The Las Cruces Bureau of Land Management, Dona Ana County Sheriff's Department, and the New Mexico State Police patrol frequently, and a campground host is present within 0.5 miles of the main campground.

MAP

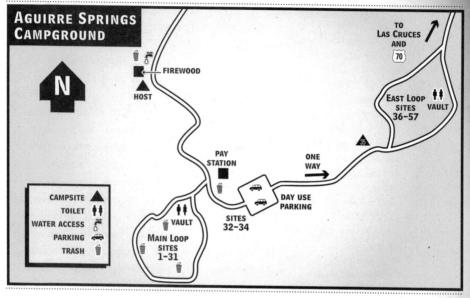

AGUIRRE SPRINGS CAMPGROUND

N

FIREWOOD

HOST

TO
LAS CRUCES
AND
70

EAST LOOP
SITES
36–57
VAULT

55

PAY
STATION

ONE
WAY

DAY USE
PARKING

CAMPSITE
TOILET
WATER ACCESS
PARKING
TRASH

VAULT

SITES
32–34

MAIN LOOP
SITES
1–31

GETTING THERE

Travel 17 miles east of Las Cruces on US 70. The turnoff is on the south side of the highway. A large sign marks the turnoff. At mile 4, the road becomes a one-way loop; travel another 2 miles to the campground. The road is paved to the campground, but drive slowly due to many of the tight turns you will encounter.

GPS COORDINATES

UTM Zone (WGS84) 13S
Easting 353152.8
Northing 353261.0
Latitude 32° 22' 15.0"
Longtitude 106° 33' 39.4"

36
PANCHO VILLA STATE PARK CAMPGROUND

> *Cacti gardens bloom from early March through the end of May.*

PANCHO VILLA STATE PARK is a campground with historical significance. This is the exact location of Camp Furlong, one of the two sites raided in 1916 by Mexican Revolutionary General Francisco "Pancho" Villa. Villa raided the camp and the tiny settlement of Columbus, a few blocks to the north. Twenty-four Americans were killed in the raid. The town of Columbus had 400 residents and was left a fiery rubble at battle's end. This is the only site since the War of 1812 in which the United States has been invaded by armed, foreign troops. Scattered throughout the grounds of the park are ruins of this once bustling U.S. Army 13th Calvary camp that housed 350 troops.

The new $1.8 million museum was dedicated in 2006 and remains free to campers. The museum contains a full-size replica Curtiss JN-3 "Jenny" airplane used by the 1st Aero Squadron. A 1915 Dodge touring car riddled with bullet holes from the raid, historic artifacts, and military weapons and ribbons can be viewed a the museum. The first armored tank ever used by the U.S. Army in battle stands as a sentinel outside the facility. The airfield was located across US 11 from Camp Furlong. The pursuit of Villa by General John "Black Jack" Pershing was unsuccessful but historic. It was the first time aircraft and battle tanks were used in combat prior to World War I.

The 49-acre park boasts indescribably beautiful cactus gardens scattered throughout the entire park. The cacti bloom from early March through the end of May, an excellent time to visit. Six ruins are worthy of photographs, so do not forget your camera. Coote's Hill is the predominate landmark of the park. It was here that under cover of darkness, the Villista raiders scouted around the north side of the hill to attack the camp. Today, Coote's Hill is beautiful, and cacti of every species thrive on the hillside. A paved walkway

RATINGS

Beauty: ✪ ✪ ✪
Privacy: ✪
Spaciousness: ✪ ✪
Quiet: ✪ ✪ ✪ ✪
Security: ✪ ✪ ✪ ✪ ✪
Cleanliness: ✪ ✪ ✪ ✪ ✪

leads to the hill's crest. You can see 100 miles on a clear day, and view nearby Palomas, Mexico, 3 miles to the south.

This Chihuahuan Desert park boasts 62 developed sites for RVs, a small grassy area for tents, plus three tent sites, C-1 through C-3, on the west side of Coote's Hill. Despite minimal tent-camping provisions, it is still excellent tent camping. The tent area has a windbreak of cottonwood and willow trees, which partition the tent area from the RV area. The grass tent area is kept watered and is perfectly level with several picnic tables and one shade shelter. The tent area is surrounded by cacti gardens and within walking distance of everything in the park. The rangers, volunteer camp hosts, and museum staff are very helpful and friendly.

Greasewood and mesquite trees dot the park. There is no firewood gathering, so bring your own. Portable fire rings are available for the asking. The modern pressurized water system delivers treated water with a strange taste unless filtered. Two modern comfort stations have sinks, flush toilets, and warm water showers, which are kept spotlessly clean. Cottontail rabbits inhabit this park in great numbers. Various bird species abound, and quail scurrying around the camp are a common sight.

Snowbirds are attracted to this park during winter months where daytime temperatures rarely plummet below the 50°F range. Summers may exceed 110°F, and there are no ponds, streams, or swimming pools in which to cool off. Spring and fall are excellent seasons to visit but windy. Campground roads are gravel, and the wind will generate a dusty camping experience.

Columbus has a museum located in the former train depot. Columbus has 700 residents, several cafes, a grocery store, and two service stations. The sleepy little border town of Palomas, Mexico, is 3 miles to the south. Shopping, restaurants, and medical and dental clinics are plentiful. Proof of U.S. citizenship is required to get back across the border. Contraband searches are performed regularly by the U.S. Border Patrol upon re entry.

KEY INFORMATION

ADDRESS:	Pancho Villa State Park
	Junction of Highways 9 and 11
	P.O. Box 450
	Columbus, NM 88029
	(505) 531-2119
	www.emnrd.state .nm.us/PRD/ PanchoVilla.htm
OPERATED BY:	New Mexico State Parks
OPEN:	Year-round
SITES:	62 developed sites, some reserveable sites; all tent sites are first come, first served
EACH SITE HAS:	Parking space, picnic table, and fire ring
REGISTRATION:	Self-service registration immediately upon selecting campsite
FEE:	$12 per night developed, $8 per night tent sites
ELEVATION:	4,064 feet
RESTRICTIONS:	*Pets:* On leash, 6-foot maximum; take precautionary measures for rattlesnakes
	Fires: Wood fires permitted only in provided fire rings; charcoal grills permitted
	Alcohol: Within campsite only
	Quiet Hours: 10 p.m.–8 a.m.
	Stay Limit: 14 days

MAP

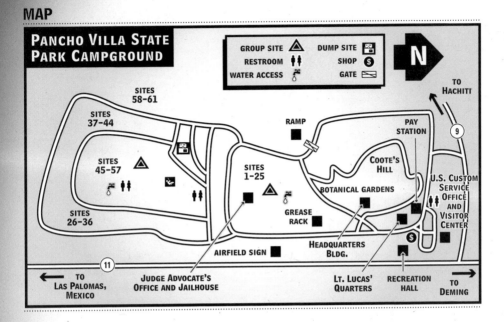

GETTING THERE

From Deming, drive 35 miles south on US 11 to the intersection of US 9. Turn west on US 9, and the park entrance is on south side.

GPS COORDINATES

UTM Zone (WGS84) 13R
Easting 0249972
Northing 3524352
Latitude 31° 49' 38.8"
Longtitude 107° 38' 30.1"

SOUTHERN NEW MEXICO
NORTHERN GILA

> *A surprisingly pretty getaway, tucked in a small box canyon*

WATER **C**ANYON **C**AMPGROUND is a surprisingly scenic getaway, tucked in a small box canyon, just 22 miles southwest of Socorro. It is an ideal family campground, with bicycle trails and one hiking trail that leads to the top of the canyon.

The Magdalena Mountains are home to black bear, coyote, mountain lion, bobcat, deer, elk, turkey, bald eagle, and several varieties of hawk. The walls of Water Canyon provide habitat for perigrine falcon and many other varieties of birds, Hummingbirds love this canyon, so bring your feeder.

The road is dirt and gravel and also quite dusty. You'll find a few tight turns on the entry road, and the loop is tight, so you will see few RVs at this camp. No campground host resides here, but the Forest Service patrols occasionally as does the New Mexico Game and Fish Department.

The forest provides great shade, with ponderosa pine, alligator juniper, pinon, and cedar trees. Most days are warm, and it is an ideal spring and fall campground, but hot in summers. You'll find plenty of downed firewood here. This canyon can get very dry, and campfire restrictions can go into effect with little notice, so calling ahead is advisable. No water is here, so bring your own, making sure you have plenty to douse your fire.

Each campsite has a fire ring and picnic table with adequate parking. There is no grass, and the ground is quite rocky, so bring a good quality ground pad. Most campsites are small and there is little privacy with the exception of trees between the sites. There are two modern wheelchair-accessible vault toilets; one at the entrance and one on the end loop with varmint-proof trash receptacles. If the trash receptacles are full, you must pack out your trash. This campground is extremely clean, kept that way by the campers, so

RATINGS

Beauty: ☆ ☆ ☆ ☆
Privacy: ☆
Spaciousness: ☆
Quiet: ☆ ☆ ☆
Security: ☆ ☆
Cleanliness: ☆ ☆ ☆ ☆ ☆

please do your part.

Just past this campground entrance is the group camp, which is used for overflow if it is not reserved. The group camp has one modern wheelchair-accessible vault toilet and a large shelter. The large grassy picnic area is located at the bottom of the hill before reaching the main campground. The picnic area has a modern wheelchair-accessible vault toilet with a large group shelter, several pedestal grills, and a small stream. The stream is usually dry unless it rains or during snowmelt.

Nearby Water Canyon's nearest supply center is the town of Magdalena. While driving down Forest Service 235, large herds of pronghorn antelope are common. This road is open range with little fencing, so be careful. Two other small campgrounds are nearby, Beartrap and Hughes Mill. The combined capacity for these two camps is eight sites.

KEY INFORMATION

ADDRESS: Magdalena Ranger District
P.O. Box 45
Magdalena, NM 87825
(505) 854-2281
www.fs.fed.us/r3/
cibola/districts/
magdalena.shtml

OPERATED BY: Magdalena Ranger District
Cibola National Forest
U.S. Department of Agriculture

OPEN: Year-round; call for road conditions during inclement weather

SITES: 12 individual sites; all sites are first come, first served; group camp used for overflow; capacity 12 sites, including several dispersed sites

EACH SITE HAS: Parking space, picnic table, and fire ring.

FEE: No fee

ELEVATION: 6,948 feet

RESTRICTIONS: *Pets:* On leash, 6-foot maximum; take precautionary measures for predators
Fires: Wood fires permitted only in provided fire rings; charcoal grills are permitted
Alcohol: Within campsite only
Quiet Hours: 10 p.m.–8 a.m.
Stay Limit: 14 days

MAP

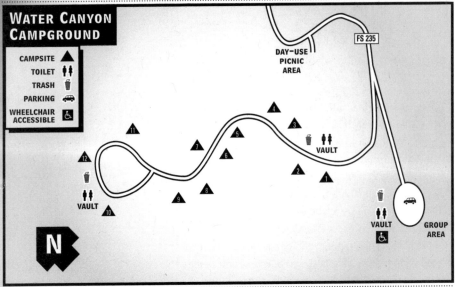

WATER CANYON CAMPGROUND

CAMPSITE ▲
TOILET
TRASH
PARKING
WHEELCHAIR ACCESSIBLE

FS 235

DAY-USE PICNIC AREA

VAULT

VAULT

VAULT

GROUP AREA

N

GETTING THERE

From Socorro, drive west on NM 60 for 16 miles, and then turn south on FS 235 at the Water Canyon sign and go 4.5 miles to the camp.

GPS COORDINATES

UTM Zone (WGS84) 13S
Easting 0303004
Northing 3766898
Latitude 34° 01' 27.3"
Longtitude 107° 08' 01.0"

38
DATIL WELL
CAMPGROUND

DATIL WELL CAMPGROUND is a historic stop for those who love the history of the Old West. Datil Well is named for the town of Datil, 1 mile to the west. This is the location of one of 15 water wells spaced 10 miles apart along the old Magdalena Cattle Trail. This trail was established in January of 1885 and stretched 120 miles from Springerville, Arizona, to Magdalena, New Mexico.

The Atchison, Topeka, and Santa Fe Railway completed its line from Magdalena to Soccoro, and ranchers began driving their livestock to Magdalena for shipment. The trail was set aside by the U.S. Department of the Interior in 1918 as a result of the Endangered Grazing Homestead Act. 1919 was the peak year of use of the trail when 150,000 sheep and 21,667 cattle made the journey.

The campground is scenic and shaded with a mix of juniper and pinon trees. Most campsites are rather small, but plenty of trees between sites provide adequate privacy. Five water hydrants are spread equally throughout the campground, delivering water from the same source used in the cattle drives. The water is treated with chlorine and should be filtered before drinking.

Three modern vault toilets are scattered conveniently throughout the campground, and one is wheelchair accessible. A friendly campground host is on-site, and there is a treasure of information and brochures at the pay station building. No special area exists for tents. RVs do use this campground and are allowed the use of generators.

All sites are ideal for tents. The ground is level with a mix of fine gravel and sand. There is no grass. The sites on the outside of the loop provide more shade and separation from the other sites and come with a view of the surrounding San Augustin plains.

> *A historic stop along the old Magdalena Cattle Trail*

RATINGS

Beauty: ☆ ☆ ☆
Privacy: ☆ ☆ ☆ ☆
Spaciousness: ☆ ☆
Quiet: ☆ ☆ ☆ ☆
Security: ☆ ☆ ☆ ☆ ☆
Cleanliness: ☆ ☆ ☆ ☆ ☆

KEY INFORMATION

ADDRESS: Bureau of Land Management Soccoro Field Office 901 Highway 85 Soccoro, NM 87113 (505) 835-0412 www.nm.blm.gov/ recreation/socorro/ docs/Datil_Well_ Brochure_jes.pdf

OPERATED BY: Bureau of Land Management

OPEN: Year-round

SITES: 22 individual sites; all sites are first come, first served

EACH SITE HAS: Parking space, picnic table, trash can, and fire ring

REGISTRATION: Self-service registration, immediately upon selecting campsite

FEE: $5 per night single unit

ELEVATION: 7,434 feet

RESTRICTIONS: *Pets:* On leash, 6-foot maximum; take precautionary measures for predators
Fires: Wood fires permitted only in provided fire rings; charcoal grills are permitted
Alcohol: Within campsite only
Quiet Hours: 10 p.m.– 8 a.m.
Stay Limit: 7 days

This campground is open year-round, and hosts are assigned here from April until November. Winter can bring more than a foot of snow, providing an excellent winter camping experience for the more adventurous. Water hydrants are turned off in November, but water is available in Datil.

The Bureau of Land Management manages this campground well, providing each campsite a small armful of wood for a campfire, but you may wish to bring a supply of your own. There is no firewood to gather. Each site comes equipped with a picnic table, fire ring, and trash can.

Three miles of hiking trails meander throughout the nearby woodlands. Hiking trails are for foot traffic only; no bicycles or motorized vehicles are permitted access. Winter snows provide excellent snowshoeing and cross-country skiing. All hiking trails range from easy to moderate, and three overlooks provide views of Crosby Canyon and the San Augustin plains.

Since the summer of 2005, heavy rains have blessed this area with green grasses and many species of wildflowers. You will see occasional deer, coyote, and many varieties of reptiles including several species of rattlesnake. Bring the hummingbird feeder, too, because the broadtails are abundant here.

Summer temperatures can soar close to 90°F here, but evenings cool off to the mid-50s. Summer rains arrive almost daily with the New Mexico monsoon season, so be careful and take cover if lightning is present.

Fifteen miles east of Datil, the Very Large Array (VLA) comprises a series of 27 radio telescopes, spread in a Y pattern across the San Augustin plain. The VLA has been used by more astronomers than any other radio telescope worldwide.

MAP

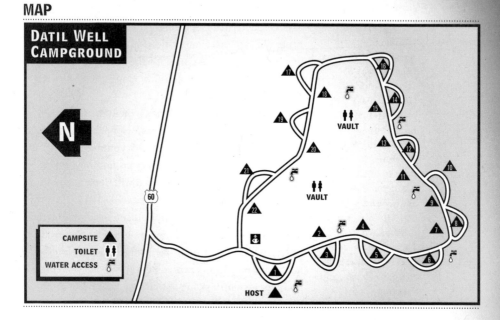

DATIL WELL CAMPGROUND

N

CAMPSITE ▲
TOILET
WATER ACCESS

VAULT

VAULT

HOST

60

GETTING THERE

From Datil Junction of US 60 and NM 12, follow US 1 mile west. Turn Left at campground sign.

GPS COORDINATES

UTM Zone (WGS84) 13S
Easting 0236494
Northing 3782941
Latitude 34° 09' 15.0"
Longtitude 107° 51' 29.3"

> *Commanding views*
> *of the lake and*
> *surrounding mountains*

PINON **C**AMPGROUND **SITS ATOP** a hill above scenic, blue Quemado Lake. This lovely campground is shaded by pinon, cedar, and juniper trees. The campground provides commanding views of the lake and surrounding mountains. Due to its location away from the lake, there is less traffic in this campground and it's more peaceful than nearby Juniper Campground.

Pinon Camp is divided into two separate areas; the road to the right leads to a huge group campground with several group shelters. The road to the left leads to the individual campsites. Twenty-two individual sites, numbered 37 through 59 are located on the left loop. The sites on the outside of the loop have more space between them, and there is some privacy between the sites, thanks to the trees.

The ground is rocky, but most campsites provide a gravel tent box. The road is crushed gravel and can get quite dusty. By setting your tent back in the trees, your sleeping quarters will escape the dust clouds of passing vehicles. Campsite tables are located too close to the road, and traffic passing at a snail's pace can coat your meals with dust.

Each site comes equipped with a fire grate, pedestal grill, and picnic table. There are no electrical sites here, and the design of this campground is predominately intended for tent camping. There were no RVs here during my stay in May of 2007.

Two composting toilets are at each end of the campground. Trash receptacles and water spigots are located next to the toilet buildings. The water is purified with chlorine, so filtering is wise.

The campground is really secure; Forest Service employees are working at this campground constantly. The Catron County Sheriff's Department and Forest

RATINGS

Beauty: ✿ ✿ ✿
Privacy: ✿ ✿
Spaciousness: ✿ ✿ ✿
Quiet: ✿ ✿ ✿ ✿
Security: ✿ ✿ ✿ ✿ ✿
Cleanliness: ✿ ✿ ✿ ✿ ✿

Service law enforcement officers keep a close eye on the campground.

It is recommended you bring your own firewood or gather wood near the El Caso Campground areas. A campground host sells wood for $5 per bundle.

El Caso Campgrounds are partially developed campgrounds located at the east end of Quemado Lake, 0.5 miles east of Pinon Campground. These areas are nestled in a valley surrounded by ponderosa pine and cottonwood trees, which offer excellent shade, camping is free.

KEY INFORMATION

ADDRESS: Quemado Ranger District
P.O. Box 158
Quemado, NM 87829
(505) 773-4678
www2.srs.fs.fed.us/ r3/gila/recreation/ reccampdet.asp

OPERATED BY: Quemado Ranger District
Gila National Forest, shared responsibility with Apache National Forest

OPEN: Official season, May 1– September 30

SITES: 22 individual sites; all sites are first come, first served

EACH SITE HAS: Parking space, picnic table, pedestal grill, and fire ring

REGISTRATION: Self-service registration, immediately upon selecting campsite

FEE: $10 per night single unit

ELEVATION: 7,862 feet

RESTRICTIONS: *Pets:* On leash, 6-foot maximum
Fires: Wood fires permitted only in provided fire rings and pedestal grills; charcoal grills are permitted
Alcohol: Within campsite only
Quiet Hours: 10 p.m.– 8 a.m.
Stay Limit: 14 days

MAP

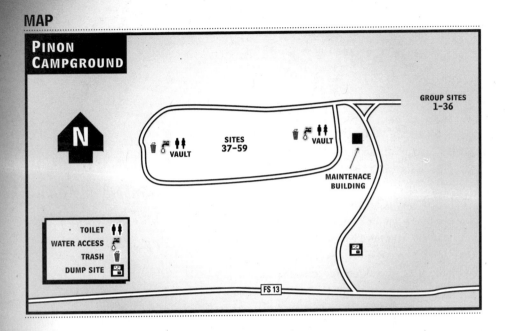

PINON CAMPGROUND

N

SITES 37–59

VAULT

VAULT

GROUP SITES 1–36

MAINTENACE BUILDING

- TOILET
- WATER ACCESS
- TRASH
- DUMP SITE

FS 13

GETTING THERE

West of Quemado take NM 32 south 14.2 miles to Quemado Lake/NM 103 sign. At the sign, turn left onto NM 103 and go 4 miles to where Forest Service 13 (gravel) begins. Continue straight on FS 13 for 1.4 miles to the campground sign. Turn left into campground.

GPS COORDINATES

UTM Zone (WGS84) 12S
Easting 0732096
Northing 3780185
Latitude 34° 08' 12.4"
Longtitude 108° 28' 58.7"

40
JUNIPER
CAMPGROUND

FOR THOSE WHO LOVE LAKE camping, Quemado Lake offers several good campgrounds. The closest camp to the lake is Juniper Campground. This is not lakeshore camping.

The fishing here can be excellent with rainbow and lake trout the most common catch, along with an occasional tiger muskie. The lake is small; 130 water acres. The lake provides two boat access ramps. Quemado Lake is excellent for canoeing, kayaking, and rafting. Personal flotation devices are mandatory while upon the water. Boats are required to travel at trolling speeds only; this is a no-wake lake. New Mexico Game and Fish wardens patrol frequently, so keep your fishing license with you at all times.

The campground sits atop a knoll above the lake and gives partial views of the lake. Most campsite views of the lake are obscured by juniper, pinon, and a few ponderosa pines. Several trails lead to the lake, less than 100 feet away. Road noise is a problem at this campground from Forest Service 13, which is located up the hill from the camp.

The campground provides 36 spaces; sites 1 through 18 are designated for RV camping and are on a separate loop from the tent area. The tent area, sites 19 through 36, is quite large. Unfortunately a few RVs will camp here, but there are plenty of sites where the parking spaces are too small for RV parking.

Tents can be erected under the trees with excellent shade. There are no grassy areas, and the ground is rocky in some spots, so bring a quality ground pad. Most sites are level, and several sites provide a tent box filled with gravel. Dust clouds are generated from the gravel road, even when vehicles drive slowly. A picnic table and fire ring is provided at each campsite and are placed close to the road.

You'll find two new, self-composting toilets, one at the loop entrance and the other at the end of the loop.

> *Excellent fishing for rainbow and lake trout and occasional tiger muskie*

RATINGS

Beauty: ✿ ✿ ✿ ✿
Privacy: ✿ ✿
Spaciousness: ✿ ✿ ✿
Quiet: ✿ ✿
Security: ✿ ✿ ✿ ✿ ✿
Cleanliness: ✿ ✿ ✿ ✿ ✿

ADDRESS: Quemado Ranger District
P.O. Box 158
Quemado, NM 87829
(505) 773-4678
www2.srs.fs.fed.us/ r3/gila/recreation/ reccampdet.asp?id=6

OPERATED BY: Quemado Ranger District
Gila National Forest, shared responsibility with Apache National Forest

OPEN: Official season, May 1–November 1

SITES: 36 individual sites; all sites are first come, first served

EACH SITE HAS: Parking space, picnic table, and fire ring, several with gravel tent boxes and pedestal grills

REGISTRATION: Self-service registration, immediately upon selecting campsite

FEE: $10 per night single unit

ELEVATION: 7,693 feet

RESTRICTIONS: *Pets:* On leash, 6-foot maximum
Fires: Wood fires permitted only in provided fire rings; charcoal grills are permitted
Alcohol: Within campsite only
Quiet Hours: 10 p.m.– 8 a.m.
Stay Limit: 14 days

Trash bins and pressurized water spigots are located near the toilets. Two other spigots, one pressurized and one hand pump spigot, are located on the loop. Because the water is treated with chlorine, it is recommended you filter the water before drinking. Bathing, cleaning pots and pans, and cleaning fish are strictly prohibited at the spigot areas. Showers are not provided at the campground.

One campground host is always assigned to the RV loop. There is no downed wood here, but the host sells firewood. The Forest Service, New Mexico game wardens, and the Catron County Sheriff's Department patrol frequently, so this campground is extremely safe. Watch children near the roadways and, obviously, at water's edge.

MAP

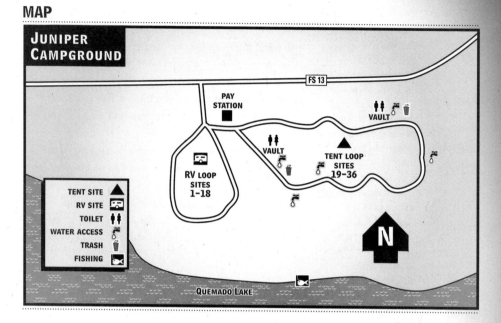

JUNIPER CAMPGROUND

FS 13

PAY STATION

VAULT

VAULT

TENT LOOP SITES 19-36

RV LOOP SITES 1-18

TENT SITE
RV SITE
TOILET
WATER ACCESS
TRASH
FISHING

N

QUEMADO LAKE

GETTING THERE

From Quemado, follow NM 32 south for 14 miles, turn east onto FS 13, and go 4 miles to the camp.

GPS COORDINATES

UTM Zone (WGS84) 12S
Easting 0731541
Northing 3780290
Latitude 34° 087' 16.3"
Longtitude 108° 09' 20.3"

41
DIPPING VAT CAMPGROUND AT SNOW LAKE

> *The cold water lake is surrounded by mountains and lush green meadows.*

WHILE DRIVING IN THE GILA WILDERNESS, my wife Susan made the comment, "God has kissed New Mexico, and New Mexico is smiling!" The rains of 2006 and 2007 have brought this lovely mountain wilderness back to health after a long era of drought. Panoramas of lush green ponderosa, fir, spruce, and oak forests greet you with meadows filled with wildflowers of many colors.

The last 8 miles along Forest Service 142 before reaching Snow Lake take you through the horrible destruction of the Bear Fire, which started June 19, 2006. A campfire out of control was blamed for the devastation. The Bear Fire consumed more than 55,000 acres and raged for more than three weeks. Dipping Vat Campground was spared as the fire stopped at the western boundary of the camp.

Snow Lake is only 100 water acres at full capacity, but it is beautiful. The lake is surrounded by mountains and lush green meadows. Rainbow trout are stocked here in early spring, summer, and late fall. Snow Lake receives excellent fishing reviews and allows boats with electric trolling motors. This is an excellent lake for canoeing, kayaking, and inflatable watercraft. The water is cold, and swimming is prohibited.

The lake has two wheelchair-accessible vault toilets, trash receptacles, a wheelchair-accessible fishing pier, a concrete boat ramp, and a large gravel parking lot. Horse trailers are permitted use of the parking lot, but pack animals are not allowed in the campground.

Have your fishing license with you at all times because New Mexico Game and Fish conservation officers patrol frequently and assist the Forest Service with

RATINGS

Beauty: ☆ ☆ ☆ ☆ ☆
Privacy: ☆ ☆ ☆ ☆
Spaciousness: ☆ ☆ ☆ ☆ ☆
Quiet: ☆ ☆ ☆ ☆ ☆
Security: ☆ ☆ ☆ ☆
Cleanliness: ☆ ☆ ☆ ☆ ☆

campground security. No campground host is assigned here.

Dipping Vat Campground sits a short walk uphill from the lake. Forty campsites are contained within two large loops. All sites offer deep grass and are excellent for tents. RV camping is restricted to vehicles under 19 feet in length, and bumpy forest roads discourage most RVs. Plenty of firewood is available within the campground.

Campsites numbered 1 through 21 are on a knoll overlooking the lake and have sparse shade. Campsites numbered 22 through 40 sit back farther, fully shaded under a canopy of mature ponderosa pines. Each site offers a concrete picnic table, fire ring, and pedestal grill. The sites are surprisingly large, which is a plus for privacy.

Four pressurized spigots provide water that should be filtered. Three modern, wheelchair-accessible vault toilets are evenly spaced throughout the campground and kept spotlessly clean. Eight varmint-proof trash receptacles are spaced throughout the camp.

Warning signs are posted for bears as well as other wildlife. Last year a pet was attacked by a fox, which was later captured and destroyed; the fox was rabid. Mexican gray wolves have been spotted in the Snow Lake vicinity. A significantly sized wolf pack resides east of Snow Lake near Loco Mountain. Howling wolves can occasionally be heard at Dipping Vat Campground. During my visit, I was not that fortunate.

On March 29, 1998, captive-reared Mexican gray wolves were released to the wild for the first time in the Blue Range Wolf Recovery Area, which includes the Gila Wilderness. The goal was a population of 100 animals. Cattlemen protested when the wolves wreaked havoc upon livestock. Twelve wolves were hunted and destroyed by the U.S. Fish and Wildlife Service in 2006. More than 25 wolves have been illegally killed by ranchers or poachers between 1998 through 2006. It is estimated that 25 to 30 Mexican gray wolves remain in the Gila National Forest.

KEY INFORMATION

ADDRESS: Reserve Ranger District
P.O. Box 170
Reserve, NM, 87830
(505) 533-6232
www2.srs.fs.fed.us/ r3/gila/about/ distmain.asp? district=reserve

OPERATED BY: Reserve Ranger District in cooperation with New Mexico Game and Fish Gila National Forest

OPEN: Official season, April 1–November 1, depending on weather; call for road conditions.

SITES: 40 individual sites; all sites are first come, first served

EACH SITE HAS: Parking space, picnic table, fire ring, pedestal grill

REGISTRATION: Self-service registration upon arrival

FEE: $5 per night

ELEVATION: 7,444 feet

RESTRICTIONS: *Pets:* On leash, 6-foot maximum; take precautionary measures for predators
Fires: Call for fire restrictions during arid seasons; fires permitted in fire rings and pedestal grills; charcoal grills permitted
Alcohol: At site
Quiet Hours: 10 p.m.– 8 a.m.
Stay Limit: 14 days

MAP

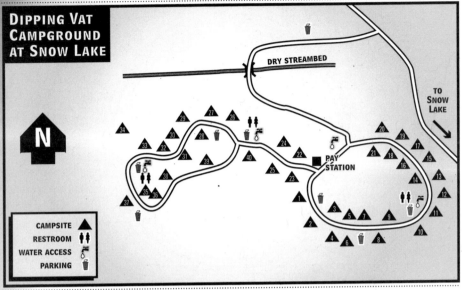

DIPPING VAT CAMPGROUND AT SNOW LAKE

DRY STREAMBED

TO SNOW LAKE

N

PAY STATION

CAMPSITE
RESTROOM
WATER ACCESS
PARKING

GETTING THERE

From Reserve, take NM 435 south until the pavement ends. This gravel road becomes FS 141. Follow FS 141 past South Fork Negrito Campground to intersection of FS 28. Turn south on FS 28, take FS 142 to the campground.

GPS COORDINATES

UTM Zone (WGSS84) 12S
Easting 0732360
Northing 3700982
Latitude 33° 25' 23.0"
Longtitude 108° 30' 03.4"

SOUTHERN NEW MEXICO
SOUTHERN GILA

42
IRON CREEK CAMPGROUND

> *Beautiful, with plenty of grass, varieties of wildflowers, and lots of shade*

IRON **C**REEK **C**AMPGROUND **IS THE FIRST** campground west of Kingston, New Mexico, along NM 152. Iron Creek is a roadside campground, and although there will be some highway noise, the view of the highway is partially blocked by tall cottonwood and willow trees along Iron Creek, which flows parallel to the highway.

The access road is paved and very appealing to tent campers, although an occasional RV will take refuge here. The tent sites provide good distance away from the campground parking for privacy, and most of the sites are large. Iron Creek is the largest campground on NM 152, with 12 campsites plus several dispersed tent areas in a mature forest, with ponderosa pine, spruce, fir, and cottonwood trees. This campground is beautiful, with plenty of grass, a variety of wildflowers, and lots of shade. The tent areas are on a terraced hill, but you'll find many level areas to pitch your tent away from the camp road.

There are two modern vault toilets, one located at the entrance road and a second located on the west loop. Each tent site has its own fire ring and picnic table. Three other tent sites have rock fire rings but no tables. Iron Creek has no host, and there is no water. The area has been picked clean of firewood, so bring your own.

The east loop has a large private campsite. This site is large enough to accommodate up to four or five large tents and is ideal for a large family group camp. For one tent it could be considered a "honeymoon suite."

Iron Creek is a bird-watcher's paradise with frequent visits by hummingbirds, so bring your feeder. Chipmunks and squirrels are seen frequently. Predators such as coyote, black bear, bobcat, and occasional mountain lion are common to this area, so keep your camp clean and put away all food items when not in

RATINGS

Beauty: ✩ ✩ ✩ ✩
Privacy: ✩ ✩ ✩ ✩
Spaciousness: ✩ ✩ ✩ ✩ ✩
Quiet: ✩ ✩
Security: ✩
Cleanliness: ✩ ✩ ✩ ✩

use. This is a campground where cleanliness is the responsibility of the user. When the refuse bins fill up, the policy is "pack it in, pack it out." Refuse pickup here is from April through October. Security is fair with occasional patrols by the Forest Service and the Sierra County Sheriff's Department.

Trail 79 is nearby, and treks for 3.5 miles to 9,991-foot-high Hillsboro Peak. Hillsboro Peak has an old log cabin, erected by the Forest Service in the 1920s and a 49-foot-high fire tower. Several miles to the west, other trails from Railroad Canyon Campground lead to the Aldo Leopold Wilderness area.

Railroad Canyon, a small campground 1 mile to the west, has four fire rings and picnic tables plus four other primitive sites with rock fire rings. There is one vault toilet and trash receptacle at this camp, which is tucked behind a high hill and therefore sheltered from road noise. The entrance road is steep, recommended for trucks or SUVs with reasonable ground clearance. Passenger cars and RVs are discouraged.

KEY INFORMATION

ADDRESS: Silver City Ranger District
3005 E. Camino del Bosque
Silver City, NM 88061
(505) 388-8201
www2.srs.fs.fed.us/r3/gila/recreation/reccampdet.asp

OPERATED BY: Silver City Ranger District, Gila National Forest

OPEN: Official season, Memorial Day–Labor Day

SITES: 12 individual sites, 3 dispersed sites; all sites are first come, first served

EACH SITE HAS: Parking space, picnic table, and fire ring

FEE: Free

ELEVATION: 7,202 feet

RESTRICTIONS: *Pets:* On leash, 6-foot maximum; take precautionary measures for predators
Fires: Wood fires permitted only in provided fire rings; charcoal grills permitted
Alcohol: Within campsite only
Stay Limit: 14 days

MAP

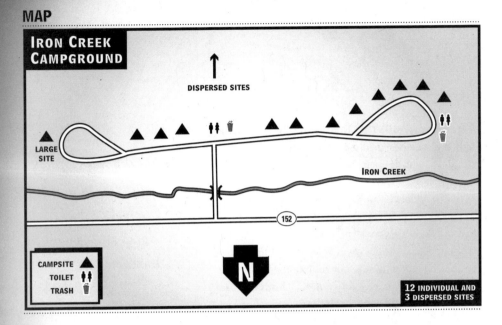

IRON CREEK CAMPGROUND

DISPERSED SITES

LARGE SITE

IRON CREEK

152

CAMPSITE
TOILET
TRASH

N

12 INDIVIDUAL AND **3** DISPERSED SITES

GETTING THERE

From Kingston, drive northeast on NM 152 10 miles; the campground sign is on the north side of the highway.

GPS COORDINATES

UTM Zone (WGS84) 13S
Easting 0237784
Northing 3644742
Latitude 32° 54' 34.2"
Longtitude 107° 48' 13.2"

43
CITY OF ROCKS
STATE PARK

MANY SOUTHERN NEW MEXICO state parks are designed more for RV enthusiasts than tent campers, but the 1,280-acre City of Rocks State Park is an exception. This park, set among gigantic boulders (some more than 50 feet high), is a geological wonder. The rock outcroppings are set in a field of tall prairie grass, with occasional mesquite, scrub oak, yucca, and various cacti. To describe this place in words cannot do it justice, nor can photographs—you just have to experience it for yourself. This is tent camping at its finest in the high-desert environment of The Mimbres Valley.

Pottery shards, arrowheads, and stone tools found here indicate Mimbres Apache tribes inhabited this area between AD 950 and 1200. Several recovered artifacts offer evidence of Spanish conquistadors passing through between 1600 and 1700. Cowboys punched cattle through this area in the 1800s, and in 1953, the movie *The Tall Texan* was filmed here. The state of New Mexico acquired the land and dedicated City of Rocks State Park in 1956.

Campsites are named after stars, planets, constellations, and galaxies. The interpretive signs at the entrance and the displays in the visitor center teach guests about the solar system. The park is an excellent place for stargazing, so bring your telescope and star chart. The stars are brilliant here, with no city lights obstructing the night sky. City of Rocks was the first state park to receive an observatory. The observatory is equipped with a 14-inch Meade LX-200 Telescope. The entire facility is solar powered, and plans are underway to include a monitor that projects images transmitted through the telescope.

Most campsites are private and set among the boulders, which quells the sounds and activities of other campers. All campsites have a picnic table and

> *Set among gigantic boulders, some over 50-feet high, City of Rocks is a geological wonder.*

RATINGS

Beauty: ✩ ✩ ✩ ✩
Privacy: ✩ ✩ ✩ ✩ ✩
Spaciousness: ✩ ✩ ✩ ✩
Quiet: ✩ ✩ ✩ ✩ ✩
Security: ✩ ✩ ✩ ✩ ✩
Cleanliness: ✩ ✩ ✩ ✩ ✩

ADDRESS: City of Rocks
State Park
NM 61, Milepost 3
P.O. Box 54
Faywood, NM 88034
(505) 536-2800
www.emnrd.state.nm
.us/PRD/cityrocks

OPERATED BY: New Mexico State
Parks Department

OPEN: Year-round

SITES: 44 developed sites
are first come, first
served; 1 group site
accommodates 35
tents; 10 RV sites can
be reserved and
offer electricity and
water

EACH SITE HAS: Parking space, picnic
table, and fire ring

REGISTRATION: Pay at visitor center
(office hours are
Monday–Saturday,
8 a.m.–5 p.m.)
or self-service
registration upon
selecting campsite

FEE: $10 per night

ELEVATION: 5,218 feet

RESTRICTIONS: *Pets:* On leash, 6-foot
maximum strictly
enforced; take
precautionary
measures for snakes,
bobcat, and coyote.
Fires: Restrictions
may be in effect
during dry seasons;
otherwise, wood
fires permitted only
in provided fire
rings; charcoal grills
permitted
Alcohol: Within
campsite only
Quiet Hours: 10 p.m.–
8 a.m. (strictly
enforced)
Stay Limit: 14 days

fire grate. Boulders and juniper and desert willow trees provide surprisingly good shade. Most campsites are level, and water runoff is excellent during the rainy season. Tenters can pitch tents on the gravel areas provided or between boulders. Nearly all sites have trash bins.

The RV area has ten powered sites with electricity and water spigots. RVs are allowed to use nonpowered sites, but parking is too difficult and not level at most sites. Generators are not allowed. Roads are gravel and can become quite dusty when windy. Signs mandate a 10-mph speed limit within the park. No off-road trails for ATVs or motorcycles exist in the park—all motorized traffic must remain on the roads.

Four modern vault toilets are strategically located throughout the park. They require a ten-minute walk from the farthest campsites. The well, powered by two windmills, delivers fresh, cool groundwater. The water is treated with chlorine, so filtering is wise. The visitor center has a modern comfort station with flush toilets, sinks, and solar-powered, warm-water showers. There is no firewood in the campground; you must bring your own.

A small botanical garden lies near the well at the visitor center, and a larger garden on the south loop road features cacti. Cacti begin blooming in March and continue their colorful show until mid-May. These cacti gardens are a photographer's delight.

The park features several hiking trails—mountain bikes are allowed on the trails. Rock climbing is popular here, but climb at your own risk. Supervise adventurous children, and remember that the nearest hospital is 26 miles away in Deming. Pay phones are available at the visitor center, but you won't be able to receive cellular service here.

The best camping seasons are spring and fall. Summertime can produce sweltering temperatures of more than 100°F, but evenings cool into the 70s. Winter temperatures average in the mid-50s during the day but often drop to freezing at night. November sees an increase in park visitors with the arrival of the snowbirds.

Pronghorn antelope, mule deer, wild burros, cottontail rabbits, badgers, bobcats, chipmunks, squirrels,

MAP

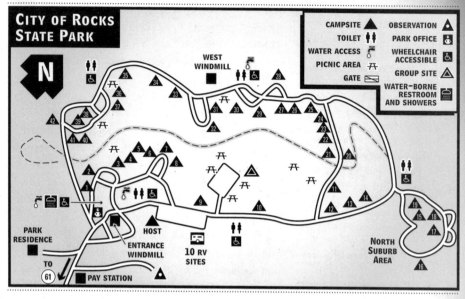

CITY OF ROCKS STATE PARK

CAMPSITE ▲	OBSERVATION △
TOILET ♦♦	PARK OFFICE
WATER ACCESS	WHEELCHAIR ACCESSIBLE
PICNIC AREA 🌲	GROUP SITE △
GATE	WATER-BORNE RESTROOM AND SHOWERS

WEST WINDMILL

PARK RESIDENCE

HOST

ENTRANCE WINDMILL

10 RV SITES

NORTH SUBURB AREA

TO 61

PAY STATION

and packrats reside here, and coyotes sing their eerie song nearly every night. More than 75 species of birds reside in the park. Box turtles and various species of lizards also call the park home. Western diamondback rattlesnakes and prairie rattlesnakes are active in the warmer seasons, especially at night. When hiking, walk cautiously and avoid wearing shorts; ankle-high hiking boots are recommended. Keep pets leashed and a close eye on your children.

Well-trained and friendly rangers supervise the park and are strict with the rules to insure a family atmosphere. Rangers are state law enforcement officers, so the security here is excellent.

Nearby, the tiny town of Faywood has a private campground with hot springs. The closest supplies and groceries are in Deming. Rockhound State Park lies 14 miles southeast of Deming and has excellent facilities and a 100-mile view. Rockhound's campground is not tent-friendly due to lack of shade and extremely rocky ground, but it's well worth a visit. Visitors are encouraged to take their treasures home.

GETTING THERE

From Deming drive north 23 miles on US 180. Turn east on NM 61 and travel 3 miles to the park entrance.

GPS COORDINATES

UTM Zone (WGS84) 13S

Easting 0220810

Northing 3609522

Latitude 32° 35' 16.9"

Longtitude 107° 58' 27.7"

44
GILA CLIFF DWELLINGS
NATIONAL MONUMENT

> *This is a "do-not-miss" attraction in New Mexico.*

IF THERE IS ONE DO-NOT-MISS attraction in New Mexico, it has to be the 533-acre Gila Cliff Dwellings. This National Monument was established November 16, 1907, by President Theodore Roosevelt.

The ancient Mogollon (pronounced Muggy-own) cliff dwellings are contained inside natural caves on a rugged sandstone cliff. The cave entrances command an incredibly beautiful view facing a vertical mesa covered with coniferous trees. Approximately 180 feet below, the trail meanders along the canyon floor and crosses over a peaceful stream gently trickling by, and then rises through a series of switchbacks to the six caves that comprise the popular archaeological site.

Caves numbered 3, 4, and 5 are fully accessible. Caves 4 and 5 are interconnected. Cave number 1 is open, with only the foundation stones of the structure intact. Cave 2 is sealed and is not accessible. Cave 6 is closed to access because there were no structures built in this cave and the ceiling is deemed to be unstable.

Mimbres Apache, Hopi, and Zuni tribes claim ancestry of the Mogollon, tracing the migration north and west from this location. Mogollon people lived in these dwellings from 1280 to no later than 1320. The site was occupied by 10 to 15 families. It remains a mystery why they abandoned the cliff dwellings after only one generation of use.

Chiricahua Apache are thought to have migrated into this area, although oral traditions of the tribe claim this has always been their homeland. Great warrior Geronimo was born in the 1820s at the headwater of the Gila River, presumably near where the east, west, and middle forks of the Gila River converge (near the visitor center). Chiricahua leaders Mangas Coloradas, Cochise, and Victorio claimed this area as home. The Chiricahua were forced from their homes and into

RATINGS

Beauty: ✰ ✰ ✰
Privacy: ✰ ✰ ✰ ✰
Spaciousness: ✰ ✰ ✰
Quiet: ✰ ✰ ✰ ✰
Security: ✰ ✰ ✰ ✰ ✰
Cleanliness: ✰ ✰ ✰ ✰ ✰

exile in Oklahoma and Florida by 1886.

The visitor center is an essential stop, with a 15-minute video of the cliff dwellings, an impressive bookshop, and souvenirs. The small museum contains artifacts from the Mogollon culture, including pottery and baskets woven from the yucca plant.

The trail to the cliff dwellings is 1 mile in length. This trail is a pleasant stroll for the first 0.33 mile, and then becomes more challenging as it gains elevation. The trail begins its incline over switchbacks to the cliff dwelling site. Allow one to two hours for the round-trip.

Be sure to carry water but no tobacco products, trail snacks, or food is allowed on the trail. This is a pack-it-in, pack-it-out trail, and there are refuse containers at the trailhead, but none on the trail. The trail fee is $3 per person. Pets are not allowed on the trail, but free kennels located behind the trailhead office building are shaded and water bowls are provided. National Park Service rangers and volunteer docents host several free, guided tours during the summer and on weekends year-round.

UPPER AND LOWER SCORPION CAMPGROUNDS

Both campgrounds are nearly identical and are conveniently located just outside of the parking lot of the cliff dwellings trailhead. The campgrounds are 0.25 miles apart. The camps are set against a cliff and adjacent to the road. All sites are walk-in and situated close to the parking lot. Each campground has one modern vault toilet and varmint-proof trash receptacles.

Upper Scorpion has ten sites, and Lower Scorpion has seven sites. All campsites are shaded, but there is little grass. Some campsites are rocky, so bring a good ground pad. Each campsite is equipped with a picnic table, fire ring, and pedestal grill. Tent campers use these campgrounds. The camps are too primitive and not configured well for RVs.

Potable water is available at the cliff dwelling trailhead. The gate opens at 8 a.m. and is locked at 6 p.m. between Memorial Day and Labor Day; and locked at 4 p.m. the rest of the year. Only campers and National

KEY INFORMATION

ADDRESS: National Park Service; Gila Cliff Dwellings National Monument HC 688 Box 100 Silver City, NM 88061 (505) 536-9461 www/nps.gov/gicl

OPERATED BY: National Park Service

OPEN: Year-round

SITES: 7 individual sites at Lower Scorpion, 10 sites at Upper Scorpion; all sites are on first come, first served

EACH SITE HAS: Parking space, picnic table, pedestal grill, and fire ring

FEE: No fee

ELEVATION: 5,716 feet

RESTRICTIONS: *Pets:* On leash, 6-foot maximum; take precautionary measures for predators
Fires: Wood fires permitted only in provided fire rings; charcoal grills permitted
Alcohol: Within campsite only
Stay Limit: 14 days

Park Service vehicles pass this way after the gates close, so you will experience peaceful evenings by your fire. The campground is safe, with park service officers patrolling the area frequently.

Firewood is available nearby, several fallen cottonwood trees near the visitor's center is an ideal gathering spot.

Down the road several miles, Doc Campbell's General Store has adequate grocery supplies, with a few camping items and souvenirs.

Due to the remoteness of this area, black bear, mountain lion, bobcat, coyote, and other predators are common, so practice clean camping habits. Be on the lookout for javelinas; there is a large population of the wild hairy boars living nearby.

Between Lake Roberts and the cliff dwellings, I spotted over 30 mule deer, with many young fawns among them. Keep your camera ready.

Be sure to fill your water before the gates are closed. Speed limits vary from 10 to 30 miles per hour, and traverse over some of the wildest and most beautiful country you will ever see. Numerous roadside parking areas provide breathtaking views of the Gila Wilderness.

Follow the signs past the visitor center to the cliff dwellings. Upper and Lower Scorpion campgrounds are well marked on the east side of the road, within 0.5 miles of the cliff dwelling parking lot.

MAP

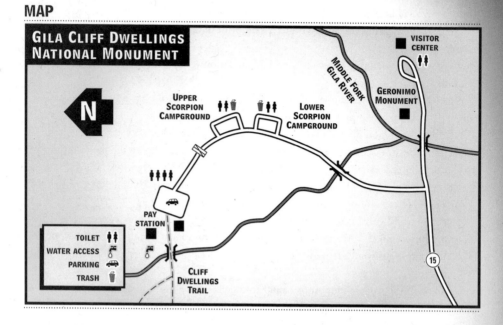

GILA CLIFF DWELLINGS NATIONAL MONUMENT

N

UPPER SCORPION CAMPGROUND

LOWER SCORPION CAMPGROUND

MIDDLE FORK GILA RIVER

VISITOR CENTER

GERONIMO MONUMENT

PAY STATION

TOILET
WATER ACCESS
PARKING
TRASH

CLIFF DWELLINGS TRAIL

15

GPS COORDINATES

UTM Zone (WGS84) 12S
Easting 0755540
Northing 3680148
Latitude 33° 13' 48.3"
Longtitude 108° 15' 28.0"

GETTING THERE

Take NM 15 north from the junction of NM 35. It is a 20-mile, 45-minute, 25 mile-per-hour drive up a narrow paved road with awesome views of the rugged Gila wilderness. The entrance to the national park is on the right. The campgrounds are located 0.5 mile farther, on the right side of the road. One mile farther is the parking lot and trail for the Gila Cliff Dwellings.

45
LAKE ROBERTS CAMPGROUNDS

> *The waters lure anglers for rainbow trout, crappie, catfish, bluegill, and bass.*

IN THE SOUTH CENTRAL GILA WILDERNESS, three lovely campgrounds provide accommodations near Lake Roberts, a 72-water-acre lake fed by the waters of Sapillo Creek. Lake Roberts is a man-made lake. Construction was managed by the New Mexico Game and Fish Department and was completed in 1963. The waters lure anglers for rainbow trout, crappie, catfish, bluegill, and bass. The nearby hamlet of Lake Roberts has one general store with a large liquor stock, ice, but very few grocery items. It is recommended you bring everything you need to avoid a 50-mile drive to Silver City, the nearest major supply center.

SAPILLO GROUP CAMPGROUND

This lovely campground is 0.25 miles south of NM 35, under a canopy of tall ponderosa pines. This primitive campground is open year-round. Sapillo Campground is used frequently as a group campground, but welcomes individual campers, space permitting. The campground has plenty of shade and level, grassy areas for tents.

The campground is situated along the highway and experiences moderate road noise. The entry road is dirt, deeply rutted in several areas, and a muddy quagmire when it rains. The surrounding area is designated as a free-range area, and cattle will be present most of the time. Please do not startle them if they are in the road.

There is one modern vault toilet, but no water or picnic tables. There are rock fire rings, but no grills are provided. There are 20 campsites, all dispersed, and camping is free.

There is no host at Sapillo, but the Forest Service and the Grant County Sheriff's Department conduct frequent patrols at this camp. Firewood is available in

RATINGS

SAPILLO
Beauty: ✩ ✩ ✩ ✩ ✩
Privacy: ✩ ✩ ✩ ✩
Spaciousness: ✩ ✩ ✩ ✩ ✩
Quiet: ✩ ✩ ✩ ✩
Security: ✩ ✩ ✩ ✩
Cleanliness: ✩ ✩ ✩ ✩ ✩

UPPER END
Beauty: ✩ ✩ ✩ ✩
Privacy: ✩ ✩ ✩ ✩
Spaciousness: ✩ ✩ ✩ ✩
Quiet: ✩ ✩
Security: ✩ ✩ ✩ ✩ ✩
Cleanliness: ✩ ✩ ✩ ✩ ✩

MESA
Beauty: ✩ ✩ ✩ ✩ ✩
Privacy: ✩ ✩ ✩ ✩
Spaciousness: ✩ ✩ ✩ ✩ ✩
Quiet: ✩ ✩ ✩ ✩
Security: ✩ ✩ ✩ ✩ ✩
Cleanliness: ✩ ✩ ✩ ✩ ✩

the surrounding forest, and the nearest water supply is at nearby Upper End Campground.

UPPER END CAMPGROUND

This popular campground is located on the eastern end of Lake Roberts. All campsites are large and well separated from neighboring campers. This camp gets extremely busy in the summer, and fills completely most weekends.

The camp sits in a mixed forest of ponderosa pine, alligator juniper, and pinon. Tent camping is excellent here, with level, grassy, shaded sites. The campground is modern; many sites are terraced with stone walls. Sites offer picnic tables, pedestal grills, and new-style fire rings.

The camp is picked clean of firewood, but there are many adjacent forest areas along NM 35 for wood gathering.

A campground host is assigned here year-round, and the camp is frequently patrolled by the Forest Service and Grant County Sheriff's Department. Fishing access is located at the loop, with a small asphalt boat ramp. The camp is equipped with two modern vault toilets and four water spigots; water should be filtered. A fish-cleaning station is located on the loop. Some road noise is noticeable from NM 35.

SITES: **12 individual sites; all sites are on a first-come, first-serve basis**

EACH SITE HAS: **Parking space, picnic table, pedestal grill, and fire ring**

REGISTRATION: **Self-service registration, immediately upon selecting campsite**

KEY INFORMATION

ADDRESS: **Wilderness Ranger District HC 68 Box 50 Mimbres, NM 88049 (505) 536-2250 www2.srs.fs.fed.us/ r3/gila**

OPERATED BY: **Wilderness Ranger District, Gila National Forest**

OPEN: **Year-round**

ELEVATION: **6,206 feet (Sapillo); 6,076 feet (Upper End); 6,160 feet (Mesa)**

FEE: **Free (Sapillo); $10 per night (Upper End and Mesa)**

RESTRICTIONS: *Pets:* **On leash, 6-foot-long maximum; take precautionary measures for predators**
Fires: **Wood fires permitted only in provided fire rings**
Alcohol: **Within campsite only**
Quiet Hours: **10 p.m.–8 a.m.**
Stay Limit: **14 days**

MESA CAMPGROUND

Mesa Campground sits atop a mesa, overlooking Lake Roberts and features pinon, common juniper, silver juniper, alligator juniper, and ponderosa pine. This campground is not just well maintained; it is manicured.

Mesa Campground is the largest of the three camps at Lake Roberts. The facilities are modern, and tent campers cohabitate well here with RVs. RV sites are on the inside of the large loop; equipped with electrical and water hookups. The sites on the outside loop are designated for tents. All spaces are shady, level, and grassy. Substantial distances between campsites ensure excellent privacy. Tent sites are large enough to accommodate three to four tents each. Restrooms are equipped with flush toilets, sinks, and electrical outlets. Outside of each restroom is a water spigot and drinking fountain. Each site has its own trash can. Firewood can be gathered along the highway outside of the camp.

SITES: 24 individual sites; all sites are on a first-come, first-served basis
EACH SITE HAS: Parking space, picnic table, pedestal grill, fire ring, and trash can
REGISTRATION: Self-service registration, immediately upon selecting campsite

GETTING THERE

TO SAPILLO
From NM 35, turn south at the campground sign and follow the road into the campground. The road can be extremely muddy. Be wary of grazing cattle.

TO UPPER END
From NM 35, turn south at the campground sign. The road leading into the camp is gravel, but the main campground road is asphalt, cutting down the dust factor.

TO MESA
From NM 35, turn south at the campground sign. The access road is paved, and parking pads are gravel.

GPS COORDINATES

SAPILLO
UTM Zone (WGS84) 12S
Easting 0769448
Northing 3656707
Latitude 33° 00' 55.9"
Longtitude 108° 06' 56.2"

UPPER END
UTM Zone (WGS84) 12S
Easting 0766108
Northing 3657959
Latitude 33° 01' 39.5"
Longtitude 108° 09' 03.4"

MESA
UTM Zone (WGS84) 12S
Easting 0765667
Northing 3658539
Latitude 33° 01' 58.7"
Longtitude 108° 09' 19.8"

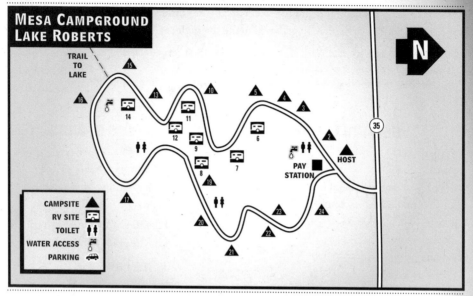

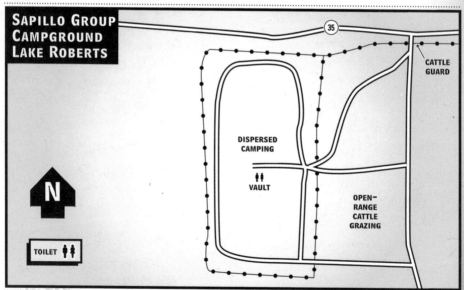

MAP

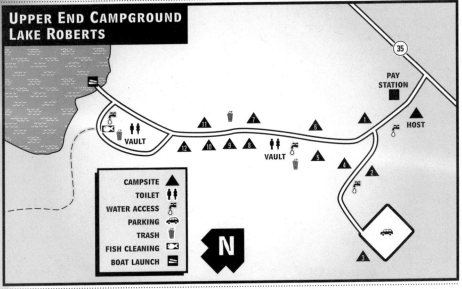

UPPER END CAMPGROUND LAKE ROBERTS

VAULT

VAULT

HOST

PAY STATION

35

CAMPSITE
TOILET
WATER ACCESS
PARKING
TRASH
FISH CLEANING
BOAT LAUNCH

N

SOUTHERN NEW MEXICO
LINCOLN

46
VALLEY OF FIRES
RECREATION AREA

> *A one-of-a-kind camping experience like no other*

AS ONE VIEWS THE Valley of Fires, one asks, "What in the heck is a Hawaiian lava field doing in the desert of New Mexico?" It is another unique joke that Mother Nature has played in the Land of Enchantment. The lava is thought to be between 2,000 and 5,000 years old (geologists are unable to agree on the age), but all agree that this is the youngest lava flow in the continental United States.

Containing both pahoehoe (pronounced puh-hoy-hoy) and aa (pronounced ah ah) lava common to the Hawaiian Islands, this incredible landscape is both eerie and beautiful. The lava flow extends for 44 miles and is between 2 to 5 miles wide along the Tularosa Valley. The lava is believed to be 165 feet thick at its deepest point. The lava field has a surface area of 127 square miles. Wildflowers, yucca, cholla, prickly pear, and many shrub species common to the Chihuahuan desert thrive here, contrasting a beautiful green hue against the brash black lava.

Valley of Fires Campground is a one-of-a-kind camping experience. The campground was originally a New Mexico State Park established in 1966. Years later, the Bureau of Land Management obtained the facility. If one word were to express this campground from a design standpoint, it would be the word text-book. The majority of the acreage is dedicated to recreational vehicles, and all RV sites have electric power, prohibiting the use of generators. A sign pro-hibits motor homes from entering the tent area.

The six site tent-camping area is shady and grassy.The tent area is shaded by juniper, pinon, and cottonwood trees. The tent sites are separated from one another by trees, scrub oak bushes, and lava boul-ders. Although the sites aren't particularly large, two tents can fit into each site. All sites have a gravel tent box and a nice grassy area to enjoy. The picnic table

RATINGS

Beauty: ✪ ✪ ✪
Privacy: ✪ ✪ ✪ ✪
Spaciousness: ✪ ✪ ✪
Quiet: ✪ ✪ ✪ ✪ ✪
Security: ✪ ✪ ✪ ✪ ✪
Cleanliness: ✪ ✪ ✪ ✪ ✪

on each site is covered by a steel shade shelter and a fire ring. Across the road from the tent sites is a modern vault toilet.

Past the tent area is a large day-use area, with a group shelter, picnic tables, pedestal grills, and a sand volleyball pit. The Hilltop Vista Overlook is a great place to catch a glimpse of the massive lava field to the north, east, and west. The entire campground can be viewed as well.

The main restroom is typical of the New Mexico State park comfort stations, roomy with flush toilets, sinks, warm-water showers, and they're kept sparkling clean. Four water spigots are available to tent campers, and all RV sites have their own water spigot. The water tastes brackish or mineral laden. Filtering may not improve the taste of this water; you might opt to bring or buy drinking water.

The 1.5-mile hiking trail leads into the heart of the lava flow, and interpretive signs identify plants, flowers, and interesting facts along the trail. Trail maps are free, and available at the visitor center. The Valley of Fires Visitor Center has books, postcards, T-shirts, and information about public lands in New Mexico. Book titles range from geology, to the history of the area, to travel guides, to plant and animal identification. Other gifts are also available.

The desert sometimes exceeds 100°F in the summer, fall, winter, and spring are wonderful times to visit. A campground host is assigned here year-round. No firewood is available, so bring your own or buy firewood in nearby Carrizozo. While in Carrizozo, try a bottle of the delicious cherry cider, taste the pecans, almonds, and pistachios, and peaches, cherries, apricots, and apples grown in nearby orchards.

KEY INFORMATION

ADDRESS: Valley of Fires Recreation Area P.O. Box 871 Carrizozo, NM 88301 (505) 648-2241 www.nm.blm.gov/recreation/roswel/valley_of_fires.htm

OPERATED BY: Bureau of Land Management, Roswell Field Office

OPEN: Year-round

SITES: 14 electrical and water equipped RV sites and 6 tent sites; all sites are first come, first served

EACH SITE HAS: Parking space, picnic table, fire ring, tent box, and shelter

REGISTRATION: Self-service registration, immediately upon selecting campsite

FEE: $18 per night RV unit; $12 per night tent site

ELEVATION: 5,710 feet

RESTRICTIONS: *Pets:* On leash, 6-foot-long maximum; take precautionary measures for predators *Fires:* Wood fires permitted only in provided fire rings; charcoal grills are permitted *Alcohol:* Within campsite only *Quiet Hours:* 10 p.m.–8 a.m. *Stay Limit:* 14 days

MAP

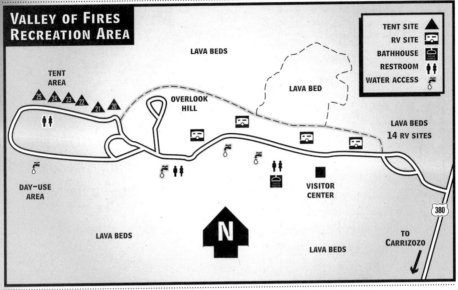

VALLEY OF FIRES RECREATION AREA

LAVA BEDS

LAVA BED

LAVA BEDS
14 RV SITES

TENT SITE ▲
RV SITE
BATHHOUSE
RESTROOM
WATER ACCESS

TENT
AREA

25 24 23 22 21 20

OVERLOOK
HILL

DAY-USE
AREA

VISITOR
CENTER

N

LAVA BEDS

LAVA BEDS

TO
CARRIZOZO

380

GETTING THERE

Valley of Fires National
Recreation Area is 4 miles
west of Carrizozo, south off
US 380.

GPS COORDINATES

UTM Zone (WGS84) 13S
Easting 0414682
Northing 3727519
Latitude 33° 41' 0.3.1"
Longtitude 105° 55' 13.7"

47
OAK GROVE
CAMPGROUND

AWAY FROM THE MADDENING CROWDS of Ruidoso, quiet Oak Grove Campground awaits just east of Alto, New Mexico. This is the White Mountain Wilderness Area, within the Sacramento Mountain Range. Here it is peaceful, wild, and uninhibited. You can enjoy the serenity of the wind in the pines and a large meadow filled with wild iris and bright green native grasses dancing in the cool mountain breezes. I awoke at 4 a.m. to the sound of a pack of coyotes singing.

Forest fire damage seen to the northwest of the camp is just one of many scars upon the mountains of Southern New Mexico. Despite the fire damage, this campground is still lovely. Sierra Blanca Peak is 3 miles from the camp as the crow flies. The campground is somewhat remote, and shaded by pinon, juniper, gamble oak, and spruce. There are 30 sites here, exceptionally well designed for tents. RVs larger than 18 feet are discouraged from the campground. The campground is private, with several campsites hidden among the rocks, with views overlooking NM 532.

There is no water, but plenty of firewood is available. There is a host's site, but it was not occupied in early June. Most of the campsites have a gravel area for the fire pit and picnic table. All sites are level, and all have plenty of shade. There are three modern vault toilets. The only downside of Oak Grove is its lack of security. There may be no host, and no Forest Service patrols were seen.

Oak Grove in the fall is an incredible campground. The oak leaves turn a fiery orange. Several herds of wild horses are native to the Sacramento Mountains. The horses often migrate to this meadow to graze. Elk are common, and their mating calls can be heard during the fall rut. Bear, mountain lion, and bobcat are common here, so keep a clean camp.

> *Wind in the pines and a large meadow filled with wild iris*

RATINGS

Beauty: ✿ ✿ ✿ ✿ ✿
Privacy: ✿ ✿ ✿ ✿ ✿
Spaciousness: ✿ ✿ ✿ ✿ ✿
Quiet: ✿ ✿ ✿ ✿ ✿
Security: ✿
Cleanliness: ✿ ✿ ✿ ✿ ✿

KEY INFORMATION

ADDRESS: Smokey Bear
Ranger District
901 Mechem
Ruidoso, NM 88345
(505) 257-4095
www.fs.fed.us/r3/
lincoln/ recreation/
d1-camping.shtml

OPERATED BY: Smokey Bear
Ranger District
Lincoln National
Forest

OPEN: Official season,
Memorial Day–
Labor Day

SITES: 30 individual sites;
all sites are first
come, first served

EACH SITE HAS: Parking space, picnic
table, and fire ring

REGISTRATION: Self-service
registration,
immediately upon
selecting campsite

FEE: $6 per night single
unit

ELEVATION: 8,745 feet

RESTRICTIONS: *Pets:* On leash; take
precautionary
measures for
predators
Fires: Wood fires
permitted only in
provided fire rings;
charcoal grills
permitted
Alcohol: Within
campsite only
Quiet Hours: 10 p.m.–
8 a.m.
Stay Limit: 14 days

A beautiful drive to the Mescalaro Tribe's Ski Apache Resort down NM 532 is a must. The road has several hairpin twists and turns and is not for the faint of heart. The views are incredible; this is the New Mexico people want to see. Elk and deer are common along the drive, so be careful.

The elevation dramatically increases from 8,400 feet at the campground to 10,066 feet at the road's summit. The road then descends to the ski basin at 9,700 foot. The summit house is 11,280 feet and the highest point of Sierra Blanca Peak is 11,549 feet. This is an incredible hiking opportunity; do not forget your camera.

Eagle Lake Campground, south of NM 532 is run by the Mescalero Apache Tribe. The camp offers fishing ponds and rustic camping with 20 sites. Nearby, Skyline Campground with 17 campsites, and the Monjeau Overlook Picnic Grounds on Forest Service 117 can be accessed by high clearance vehicles only.

MAP

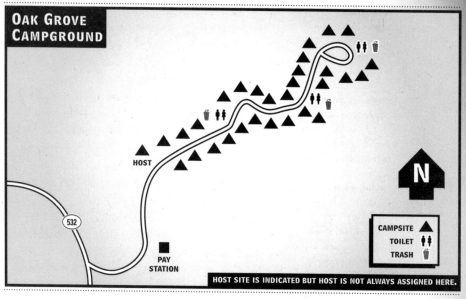

OAK GROVE CAMPGROUND

HOST

532

PAY
STATION

N

CAMPSITE ▲
TOILET ♦♦
TRASH 🗑

HOST SITE IS INDICATED BUT HOST IS NOT ALWAYS ASSIGNED HERE.

GETTING THERE

Follow NM 48 north
out of Ruidoso 4 miles,
turn west (left) on NM 532
and go 5 miles.

GPS COORDINATES

UTM Zone (WGS84) 13S
Easting 0430275
Northing 3695074
Latitude 33° 23' 33.7"
Longtitude 105° 44' 59.0"

48
SOUTHFORK CAMPGROUND

Deeply forested camp-ground adjacent to lovely Bonito Lake

SITUATED IN A CANYON at road's end just past Bonito Lake sits Southfork campground. The rugged hillside is deeply forested with ponderosa pine, juniper, spruce, fir, oak, cottonwood, and aspen trees. This campground comes alive with an array of wildflowers in spring, and they bloom all summer.

This popular campground is quite compact with 60 campsites, and you'd better plan on getting here early for a space. The best tent area is located on the right side of the road, with 16 walk-in sites numbered 1 through 16. This area is covered in tall native grasses. A restroom is located here with flush toilets and sinks. Five other vault toilets and three water spigots are placed throughout the camp.

At the end, the group camping area provides an overflow area for tent campers, provided it is not reserved. There is ample parking along the roadside. The Southfork Trail head is located at the end of the road, and there is a separate parking area for hikers.

There are two loops up the hill to the left, providing a mix of tent and RV camping. The hillside is rock and dirt, with no grass, but there are some level sites for tents. The inner loop contains campsites 18 through 40, while the outer loop sites 43 through 61. These loop areas were poorly designed. The sites are just too small and too close together. The outer loop, however, has a slight advantage because tents can be set up away from the cluster of campers providing a little more quiet. The weekend of my visit, it was so crowded that I couldn't imagine camping on the loops.

Despite the flaws of the loop sites, this campground is managed by some friendly hosts who take great pride in this campground. Weekday camping here is serene and peaceful. Weekends are madness. However, the beauty of this camp far exceeds the flaws. A bear paid a visit to the host's camp in spring

RATINGS

Beauty: ✿ ✿ ✿ ✿ ✿
Privacy: ✿
Spaciousness: ✿
Quiet: ✿
Security: ✿ ✿ ✿ ✿ ✿
Cleanliness: ✿ ✿ ✿ ✿ ✿

2007. The site was torn up pretty good, but the bear hasn't returned. On weekends, predators keep their distances due to the crowds. Frequent patrols by the U.S. Forest Service and the Lincoln County Sheriff's Department assure a safe camping environment.

Bonito Lake is owned by the City of Alamogordo, and provides its water supply. No bathing, swimming, or flotation devices are permitted in the lake. Bonito is regularly stocked with rainbow trout by the New Mexico Game and Fish Department. At the bottom of the hill is Westlake Campground, owned and managed by the City of Alamogordo. It is a huge campground, with more than 130 campsites, overcrowded, and noisy. This campground is in the process of being redesigned and will have plenty of potential in the future.

KEY INFORMATION

ADDRESS: Smokey Bear Ranger District 901 Mechem Ruidoso, NM 88345 (505) 257-4095 www.fs.fed.us/r3/lincoln/recreation/d1-camping.shtml

OPERATED BY: Smokey Bear Ranger District Lincoln National Forest U.S. Department of Agriculture

OPEN: Official season, May 15– September 15.

SITES: 60 individual sites; all sites are first come, first served

EACH SITE HAS: Parking space, picnic table, and fire ring

REGISTRATION: Self-service registration, immediately upon selecting campsite

FEE: $10 per night single unit

ELEVATION: 7,876 feet

RESTRICTIONS: *Pets:* On leash, 6-foot maximum; take precautionary measures for predators
Fires: Wood fires permitted only in provided fire ring; charcoal grills permitted
Alcohol: Within campsite only
Quiet Hours: 10 p.m.– 8 a.m.
Stay Limit: 14 days

MAP

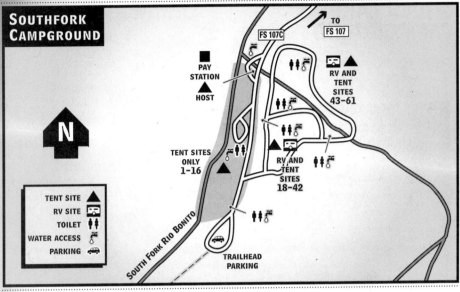

SOUTHFORK CAMPGROUND

TO FS 107

FS 107C

PAY STATION

HOST

RV AND TENT SITES 43–61

N

TENT SITES ONLY 1–16

RV AND TENT SITES 18–42

TENT SITE
RV SITE
TOILET
WATER ACCESS
PARKING

SOUTH FORK RIO BONITO

TRAILHEAD PARKING

GETTING THERE

From Ruidoso, drive North on NM 48, turn left onto US 37 for 1.5 miles, turn left on Forest Service 107 (County Road C-009), and continue 5 miles past the tiny town of Bonito and Bonito Lake about 1 mile, and turn left at campground sign.

GPS COORDINATES

UTM Zone (WGS84) 13S
Easting 0429926
Northing 3701430
Latitude 33° 27' 0.00"
Longtitude 105° 45' 14.3"

49
SILVER LAKE CAMPGROUND

FOR THOSE WHO LOVE primitive camping in a lovely setting, Silver Lake Campground on the Mescalero Apache Reservation is waiting for you. The privilege of camping on Native American land is always a thrill. It is like stepping back in time. There is no technology here, no cellular service, and no Internet access. The only link to the outside world is a pay telephone.

The Mescalero Tribe has three sub tribes; the Mescalero, the Chiricahua, and the Lipan Apache. Mescalero tribal lands encompass 720 square miles of beautiful mountain wilderness. The Mescalero business enterprises include the Inn of the Mountain Gods Resort and Casino, the Apache Nugget Casino, and the Ski Apache Resort. About 4,000 tribal members live on Mescalero land.

The friendly and helpful staff openly welcomes campers. The campground office is an A-frame cabin with a small store selling basic groceries, including ice and firewood. There is no firewood to gather within the camp.

The camp has no paved or gravel roads but is pleasant, and the surrounding mountains are beautiful. The roadways in the camp are dirt with some deep tire ruts, but there are many shady areas for tent campers under the canopy of ponderosa pines, oak, juniper, blue spruce, fir, and aspen. About 100 areas exist to pitch a tent, and it's easy to find a remote site that is level. All sites provide a picnic table and a fire ring.

RVs are not permitted in the tent area, and no tents are allowed in the RV area. All RV sites have electrical hookups, and generators are not permitted. There is a small playground in the meadow between the RV and the tent area. Each camper gets a color map of the grounds and a short list of practical campground rules. The campground is administered

> *Sleep under a canopy of ponderosa pine, oak, juniper, blue spruce, fir and aspen.*

RATINGS

Beauty: ✫ ✫ ✫ ✫ ✫
Privacy: ✫ ✫ ✫ ✫ ✫
Spaciousness: ✫ ✫ ✫ ✫ ✫
Quiet: ✫ ✫ ✫ ✫ ✫
Security: ✫ ✫ ✫ ✫ ✫
Cleanliness: ✫ ✫ ✫ ✫ ✫

KEY INFORMATION

ADDRESS: Mescalero Apache Reservation Silver Lake Campground 868 Highway 244 Mescalero, NM 88340 (505) 464-2244

OPERATED BY: Mescalero Apache Reservation

OPEN: Official season, first week of April–last week of September

SITES: 150 acres, dispersed; all sites are first come, first served

EACH SITE HAS: Parking space, picnic table, and fire ring

REGISTRATION: Register at office prior to entry

FEE: $12 per night per vehicle for 2 people, 50 cents for each additional person; check-out is 5 p.m.

ELEVATION: 7,640 feet

RESTRICTIONS: *Pets:* On leash, 6-foot maximum, strictly enforced; take precautionary measures for predators
Fires: Wood fires permitted only in provided fire rings; charcoal grills permitted
Alcohol: Within campsite only
Quiet Hours: 11 p.m-8 a.m.

similar to a private campground and is kept clean.

Mescalero police and Federal Conservation officers have jurisdiction here and assure safety. Portable toilets are distributed throughout the camp, and tent campers have their own bathhouse complete with sinks, flush toilets, and warm-water showers. Fresh water spigots are located at the entrance of the camp, and the water should be filtered.

Fishing is good here; the seven-acre lake is stocked every two weeks with rainbow trout, raised at the nearby fish hatchery, also operated by the tribe. Because this is a reservation lake, New Mexico fishing licenses are not required, and a fishing permit is $10, with a limit of five trout per permit.

MAP

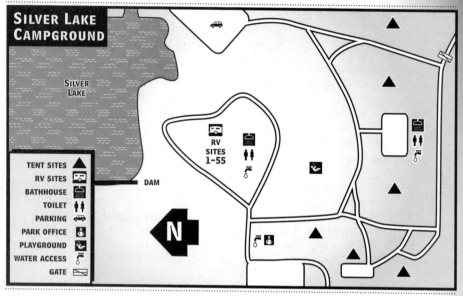

SILVER LAKE CAMPGROUND

SILVER LAKE

DAM

RV SITES 1-55

N

TENT SITES	▲
RV SITES	🚐
BATHHOUSE	🚿
TOILET	👫
PARKING	🚗
PARK OFFICE	🏢
PLAYGROUND	🛝
WATER ACCESS	🚰
GATE	▨

GETTING THERE

From Cloudcroft, take NM 82 west 1 mile, turn north on NM 244 for 8 miles. The campground is on the left side of road.

GPS COORDINATES

UTM Zone (WGS84) 13S
Easting 441249.2
Northing 3653462.2
Latitude 33° 01' 04.9"
Longtitude 105° 37' 44.7"

> *Newly renovated, a delightful tent-camper's haven*

PINES **C**AMPGROUND has to be my number one pick of all the campgrounds in Lincoln Nationa Forest. This is a delightful tent camper's haven, jsut 1.25 miles north of the town of Cloudcroft. There is cellular phone service at the campground.

Cloudcroft is a lively town of more than 700 residents. It offers two golf courses, a miniature golf course, and two astronomical observatories nearby. The Mexican Trestle, an old railroad trestle built across a steep canyon, is a popular attraction. Wireless Internet is available at the Cloudcroft Chamber of Commerce building. Mountaintop Mercantile is a full-service grocery store with camping supplies. Cloudcroft has several gasoline stations, a couple of restaurants, and an ice-cream shop and candy store for those with a sweet tooth.

Situated in a forest of mature ponderosa pine, a few spruce, fir, and gambel oak trees, Pines Campground is quite shady. All sites are on the outside of the loop, providing plenty of space between sites for privacy. The campground is more than 8,600 feet in elevation, so be prepared for cool nights, occasionally dipping into the 40°F range. The only drawback to this campground is road noise from NM 244. The highway quiets down after dark, so you will have a peaceful evening by the campfire.

This campground was completely renovated in 2006 with oiled gravel roads and parking pads. Three wheelchair-accessible vault toilets are spotless and conveniently spaced, with water spigots and varmint-proof trash receptacles. The water should be filtered, though, because the well is treated with chlorine.

Each campsite comes equipped with a new-style fire ring and picnic table. The double and triple campsites are equipped with pedestal grills. The parking pads are only large enough to accommodate 16-foot

RATINGS

Beauty: ✪ ✪ ✪ ✪ ✪
Privacy: ✪ ✪ ✪ ✪ ✪
Spaciousness: ✪ ✪ ✪ ✪ ✪
Quiet: ✪ ✪ ✪
Security: ✪ ✪ ✪ ✪ ✪
Cleanliness: ✪ ✪ ✪ ✪ ✪

trailers, and there will be a few pop-up campers. Most campsites are grassy. Showers are available at nearby Silver Campground for a $4 fee.

This campground has a host, and frequent patrols are conducted by the Forest Service and Otero County Sheriff's Department. Black bears can be common here, and it is advisable to stow all food-related items unless preparing meals or eating. You may hear coyote during the night and owls are frequently heard. Blue jays are common, as well as hummingbirds, so bring your feeders.

KEY INFORMATION

ADDRESS: Lincoln National Forest Sacramento Ranger District 1101 New York Avenue Alamogordo, NM 88310 (505) 434-7200 www.fs.fed.us/r3/lincoln

OPERATED BY: Sacramento Ranger District, Lincoln National Forest

OPEN: May 1–October 31

SITES: 48 individual sites; all are first come, first served

EACH SITE HAS: Parking space, picnic table, and fire ring; some have pedestal grill

REGISTRATION: Self-service registration, immediately upon selecting campsite

FEE: $13 per night single unit; $19 per night double unit; $25 per night triple unit; $6 per night extra vehicle

ELEVATION: 8,634 feet

RESTRICTIONS: *Pets:* On leash, 6-foot maximum; take precautionary measures for predators
Fires: Wood fires permitted only in provided fire rings; charcoal grills permitted
Alcohol: Within campsite only
Quiet Hours: 10 p.m.–8 a.m.
Stay Limit: 14 days

MAP

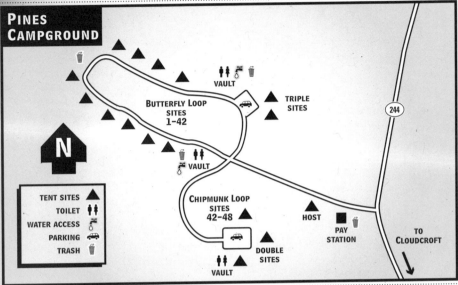

PINES CAMPGROUND

BUTTERFLY LOOP
SITES
1-42

VAULT

TRIPLE SITES

VAULT

CHIPMUNK LOOP
SITES
42-48

HOST

PAY STATION

DOUBLE SITES

VAULT

TO CLOUDCROFT

244

N

TENT SITES
TOILET
WATER ACCESS
PARKING
TRASH

GETTING THERE

From Cloudcroft, drive 1.25 miles north on NM 244. The campground turnoff is marked with a sign, to your left.

GPS COORDINATES

UTM Zone (WGS84) 13S
Easting 431297.9
Northing 364784.0
Latitude 32° 58' 0.11"
Longtitude 105° 44' 6.54"

APPENDIXES & INDEX

APPENDIX A CAMPING-EQUIPMENT CHECKLIST

Assemble a gear box and keep all your essentials packed, so you are ready to go at a moment's notice. This way all the items are in one place and will not be forgotten. You have your own camping style, and you'll know what to pack. Make a list and check it twice. The simpler you camp, the better. The following list is quite exhaustive, but will provide good ideas of what might be useful. Personal clothing, toiletries, cooler contents are for individual choice and have not been included in this list.

Prioritize your water supply. Many campgrounds profiled in this book do not have water on-site. Always carry an extra five-gallon water jug.

SLEEPING
Tent
Sleeping bag
Pillow
Ground pad
Extra blanket
Duct tape
Tent tepair tape
Rubber patch kit

COMFORT
Toilet paper
Collapsible camping chairs
Firewood
Firestarter sticks
Firelog
Lantern and extra fuel

COOKING
Campstove and extra fuel
Dutch oven
Stockpot
Sauce pan
Skillet
Utensils (knives, forks, spoons, spatula, can/bottle opener, corkscrew)
Barbecue grill lighter

Coffee pot and mugs (new style Lexan French presses work great!)
Plastic reusable plates
Paper towels
Tuffy pads (scouring pads)
Dish soap
Spices (salt, pepper, onion powder, garlic powder, beef and chicken bullion, sugar or sugar substitute packets, Parmesan cheese packets, coffee creamer packets)
Sauces (Tabasco, liquid smoke, worcestershire, steak sauce, barbecue sauce)
Nonperishable items (canned vegetables, fruit, mushrooms, green chiles, jalapeño peppers, soups, ravioli, spaghetti, chili, tamales, canned meats—easy hot lunch items)

GEAR BAG
Caribiners
Tarp(s)
Bungee cords
Rope
Rechargable batteries with car charger
Flashlights

TOOLKIT

Extra tent stakes

Extra batteries

Hand hatchet

Screwdrivers, pliers, crescent wrench, wire
   cutters, needle- nose pliers

Small roll of bailing wire

Electrical tape

Small container of nails

Collapsible shovel

Lawn rake

Full-size ax

ADVERSE WEATHER GEAR

Ball cap

Wool hat

Spare pair of shoes

Rain poncho or jacket

Gloves

Foil emergency blanket

FIRST AID KIT (Benedril, Tums, Alka
   Seltzer, cough drops, butterfly bandages,
   hydrogen peroxide, rubbing alcohol,
   compress bandages, ace bandages,anti-
   septics, scissors, single-edge razor blade,
   tweezers, hemostat, eye drops)

SAFETY

Whistle

Bear repellent

SPF sunblock

Insect repellent

Compass

Maps

Small mint tin with coins for pay telephone

FUN STUFF

Deck of cards

Favorite board games

Small battery powered DVD player with
   movies

iPod/portable CD player

Digital camera

Inflatable raft and paddles, float tube with
   powered air pump

Fishing gear, bait, and fishing license

Wildlife, birding, and flora identification
   booklets

Bird feeders

Football, Frisbees. sports items

Bicycles

APPENDIX B
SOURCES OF INFORMATION

Cochiti Lake Dam Projects Office
U.S. Army Corps of Engineers
82 Dam Crest Road
Peña Blanca, NM 87041-5015
(505) 465-0307/0308/2300
www.spa.usace.army.mil/recreation/
  cochiti/campgrounds.htm

Socorro Field Office (Datil Well)
Bureau of Land Management
901 S. Highway 85
Socorro, NM 87801-4168
(505) 835-0412; fax (505) 835-0223
www.blm.gov/nm/st/en/fo/Socorro_
  Field_Office.html

**Las Cruces District Office
  (Aguirre Spring)**
Bureau of Land Management
1800 Marquess Street
Las Cruces, NM 88005-3370
(505) 525-4300
www.blm.gov/nm/st/en/fo/Las_Cruces_
  District_Office.html

Jicarilla Game and Fish (Jicarilla Lakes)
P.O Box 313
Dulce, NM. 87255
(505) 759-3255; fax (505) 759-3457
www.jicarillahunt.com

**Mescalero Apache Reservation
  (Silver Lake)**
868 Highway 244
Mescalero, NM 88340
(505) 464-2244

Carson National Forest
208 Cruz Alta Road
Taos, NM 87571
(575) 758-6200
www.fs.fed.us/r3/carson/index.shtml

Gila National Forest
3005 E. Camino del Bosque
Silver City, NM 88061
(505) 388-8201
www2.srs.fs.fed.us/r3/gila

Lincoln National Forest
1101 New York Ave.
Alamogordo, NM 88310
(575) 434-7200
www.fs.fed.us/r3/lincoln/index.shtml

Santa Fe National Forest
1474 Rodeo Road
Santa Fe, NM 87505
(505) 438-7840; fax (505) 438-7834
www.fs.fed.us/r3/sfe/

New Mexico State Parks
1220 South St. Francis Drive
Santa Fe, NM 87505
(505) 476-3355 or (888) NMPARKS
  (667-2757)
fax (505) 476-3361
www.emnrd.state.nm.us/PRD/Index.htm

INDEX

Page references followed by *m* indicate a map.

Looking For More Info?

Menasha Ridge Press has partnered
with Trails.com to provide additional
information for all the trails in this
book, including:

- Topo map downloads
- Real-time weather
- Trail reports, and more

To access this information, visit:

http://menasharidge.trails.com

In Partnership With

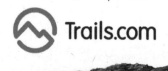

Trails.com

CHECK OUT THESE OTHER GREAT TITLES
FROM MENASHA RIDGE PRESS!

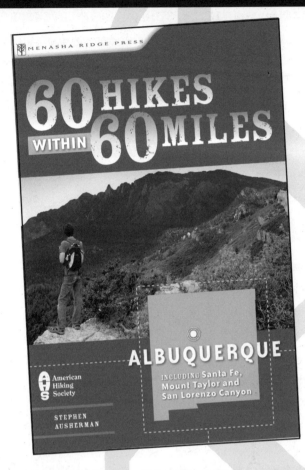

60 HIKES WITHIN 60 MILES: ALBUQUERQUE

by Stephen Ausherman
0-89732-590-7 • 978-0-89732-590-5
$16.95
6 x 9, paperback
maps, photographs, index

Hikes lead to ancient pueblos, ghost towns, slot canyons, strange hoodoos and other treasures in the heart of New Mexico, all just a daytrip or less from the Duke City.

DEAR CUSTOMERS AND FRIENDS,

SUPPORTING YOUR INTEREST IN OUTDOOR ADVENTURE, travel, and an active lifestyle is central to our operations, from the authors we choose to the locations we detail to the way we design our books. Menasha Ridge Press was incorporated in 1982 by a group of veteran outdoorsmen and professional outfitters. For 25 years now, we've specialized in creating books that benefit the outdoors enthusiast.

Almost immediately, Menasha Ridge Press earned a reputation for revolutionizing outdoors- and travel-guidebook publishing. For such activities as canoeing, kayaking, hiking, backpacking, and mountain biking, we established new standards of quality that transformed the whole genre, resulting in outdoor-recreation guides of great sophistication and solid content. Menasha Ridge continues to be outdoor publishing's greatest innovator.

The folks at Menasha Ridge Press are as at home on a white-water river or mountain trail as they are editing a manuscript. The books we build for you are the best they can be, because we're responding to your needs. Plus, we use and depend on them ourselves.

We look forward to seeing you on the river or the trail. If you'd like to contact us directly, join in at www.trekalong.com or visit us at www.menasharidge.com. We thank you for your interest in our books and the natural world around us all.

SAFE TRAVELS,

Bob Sehlinger

BOB SEHLINGER
PUBLISHER